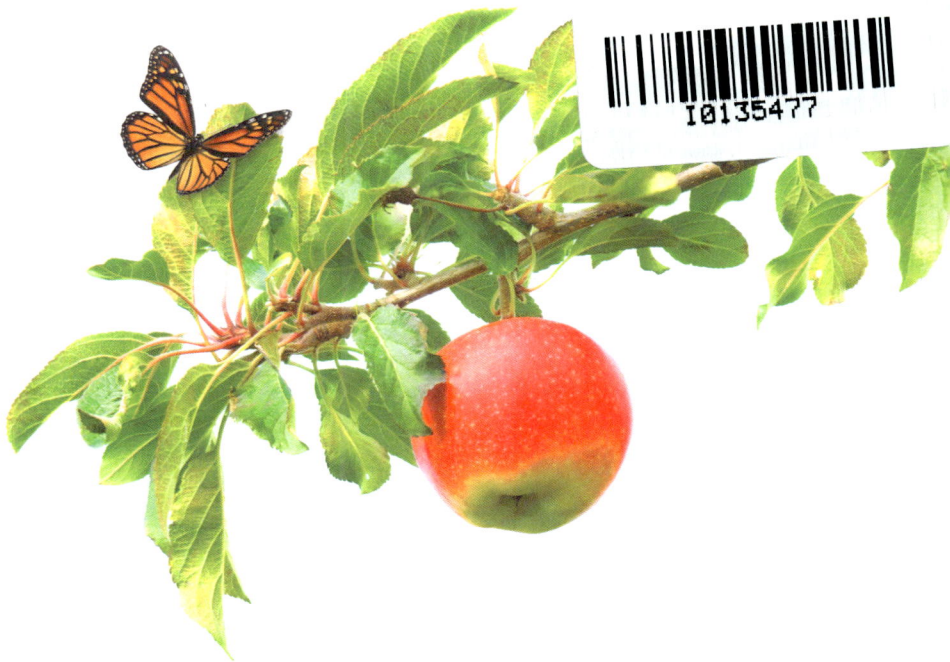

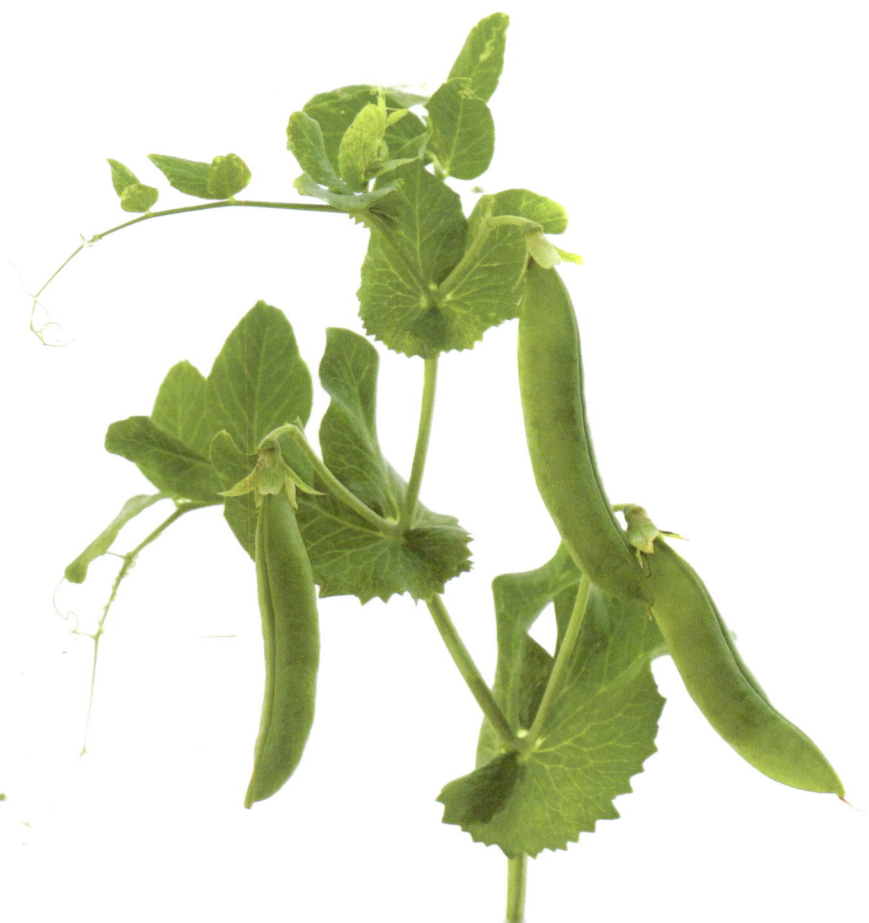

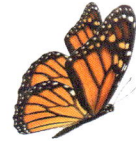

We can help create a culture – imagine this –
where our kids ask for healthy options
instead of resisting them.

Michelle Obama

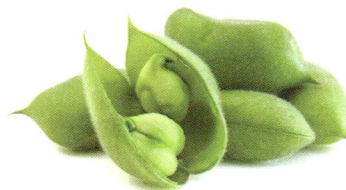

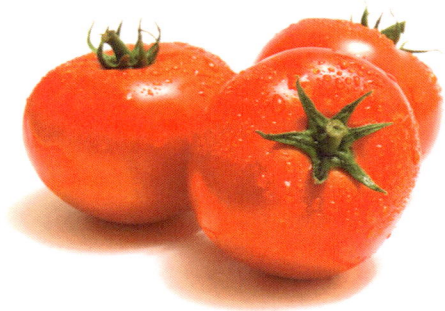

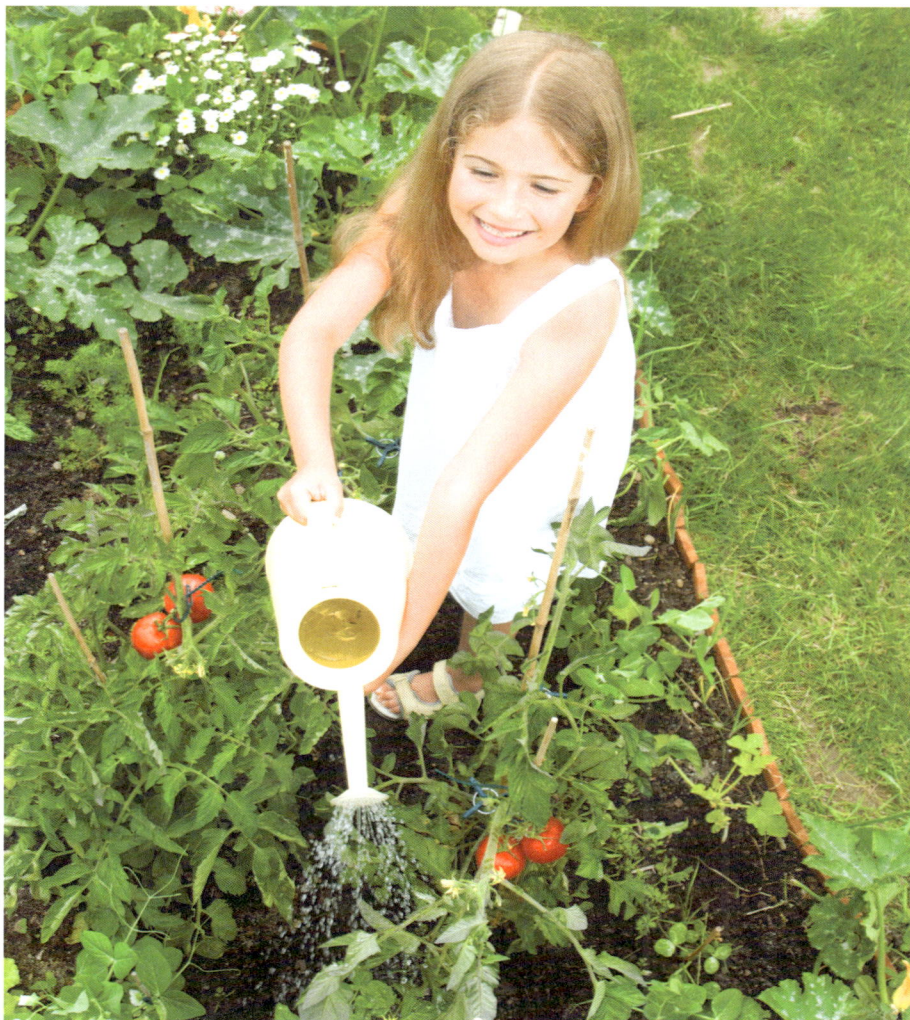

Eating Lean & Green

with Super Foods to Save the Planet!

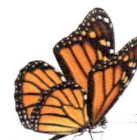

Barbara Cole Gates

A publication of Lean and Green Kids

Book design by Barbara Cole Gates.

ISBN: 978- 0-9974461-0-4
[1. Health & Daily Living, Diet & Nutrition – Juvenile nonfiction.
2. Science & Nature, Environmental Conservation and Protection – Juvenile nonfiction.]

leanandgreenkids.org

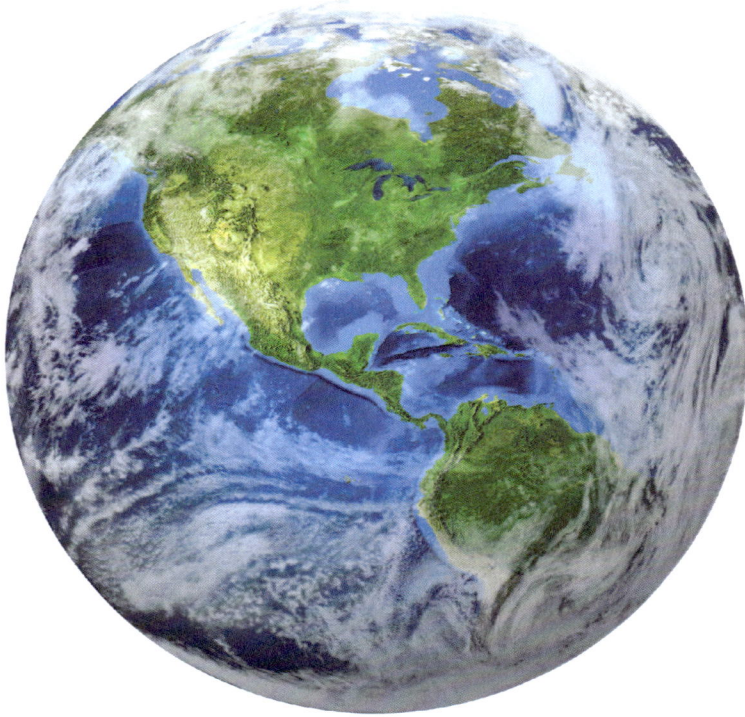

Dedicated to children around the
world who care for our precious
planet and all its creatures,
great and small.

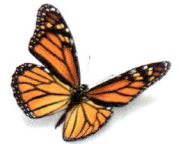

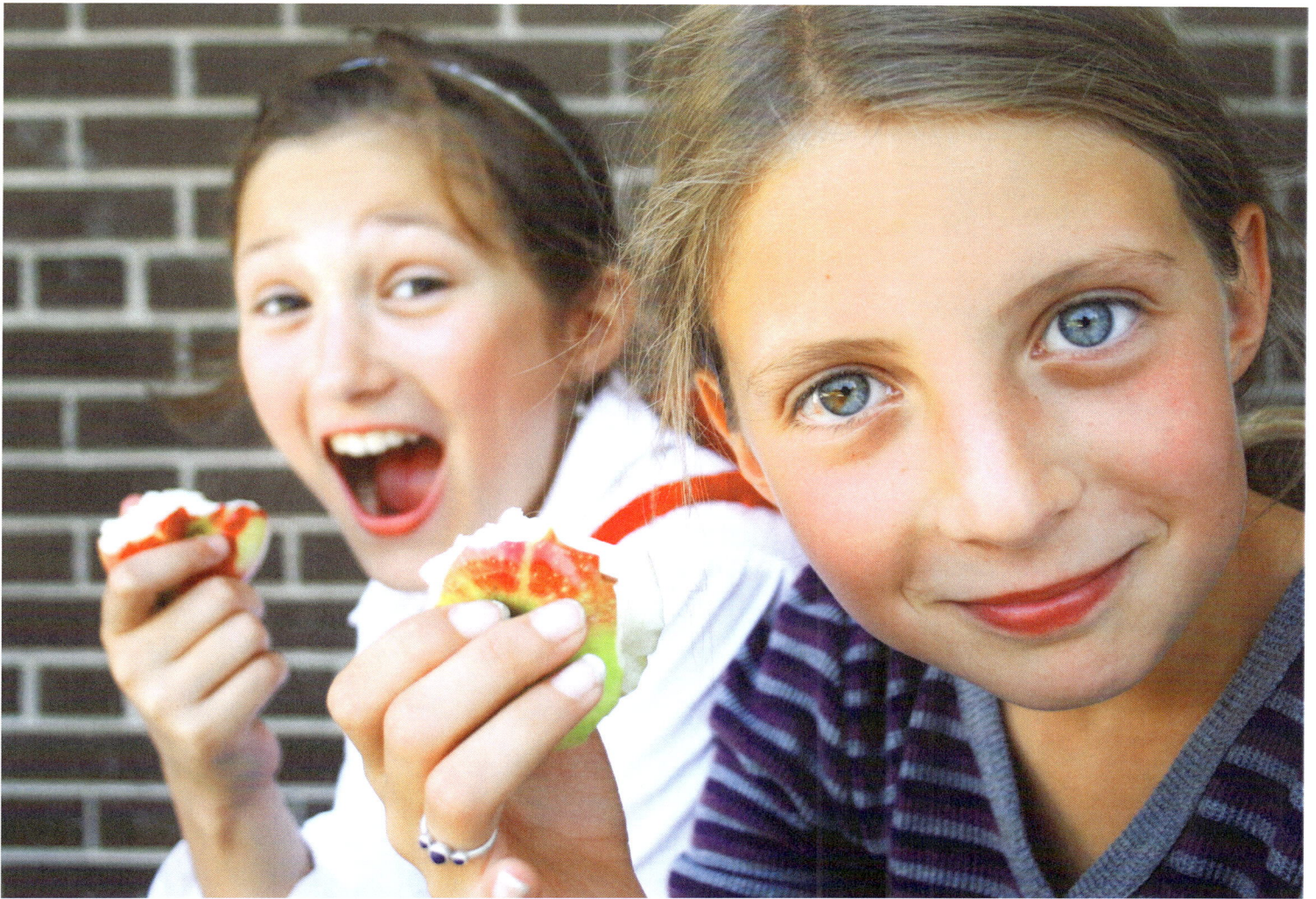

Eating.

It's something we need to do and it's something we love to do.
What to eat is one of the most important decisions of your day!

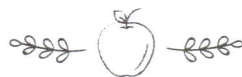

🍎

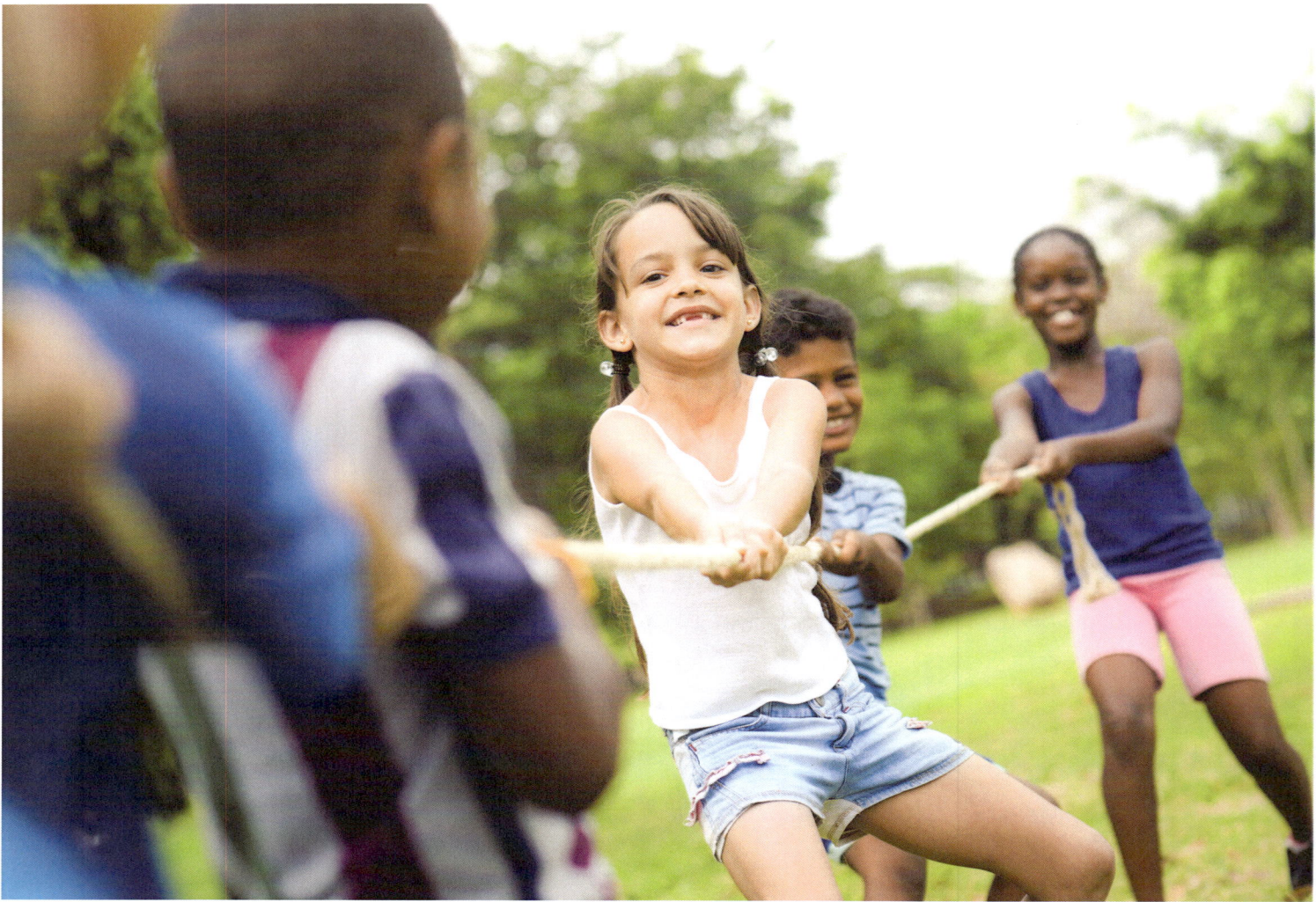

Healthy food choices help you to have a strong body,

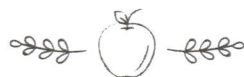

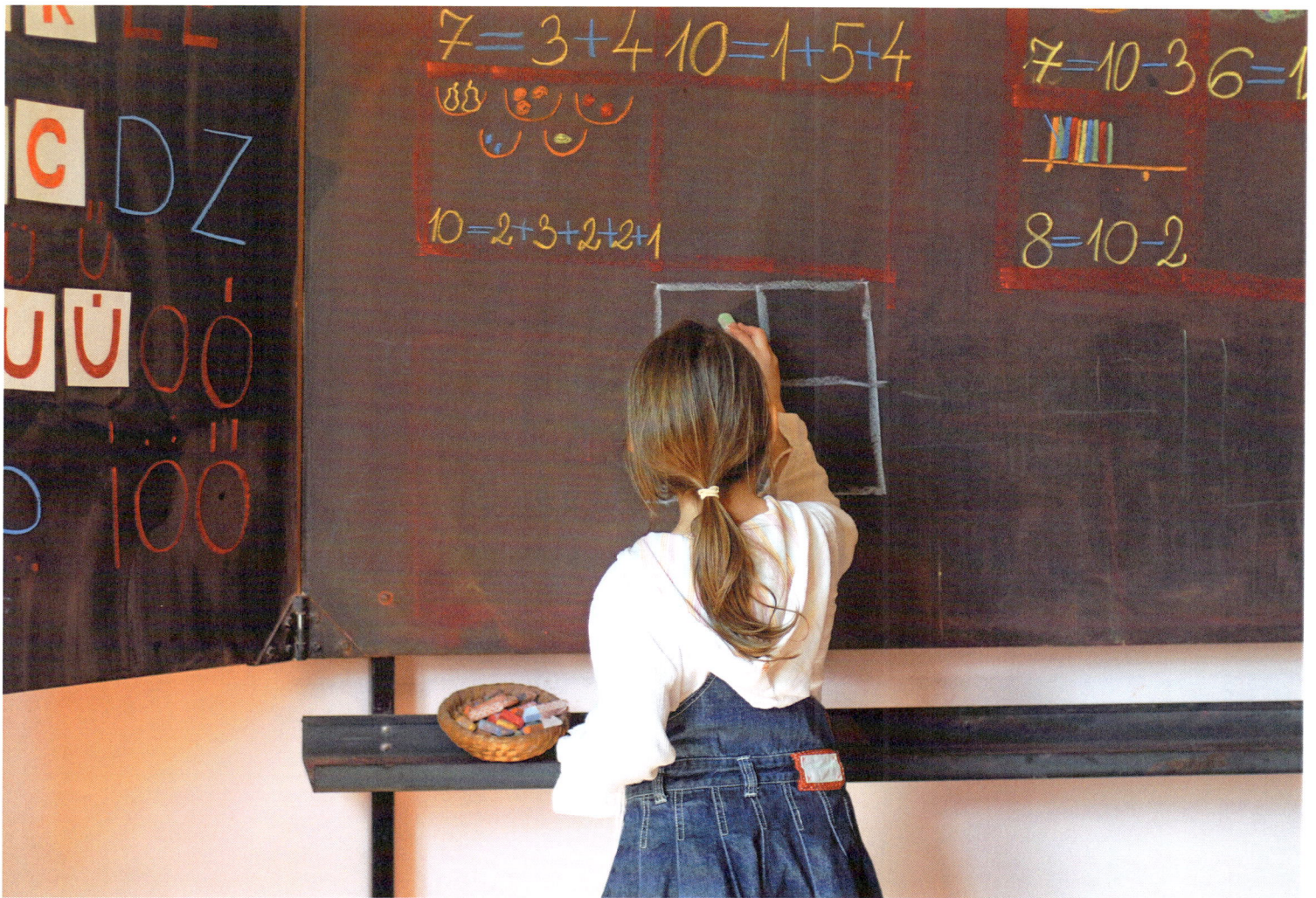

a sharp mind,

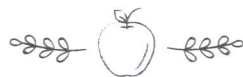

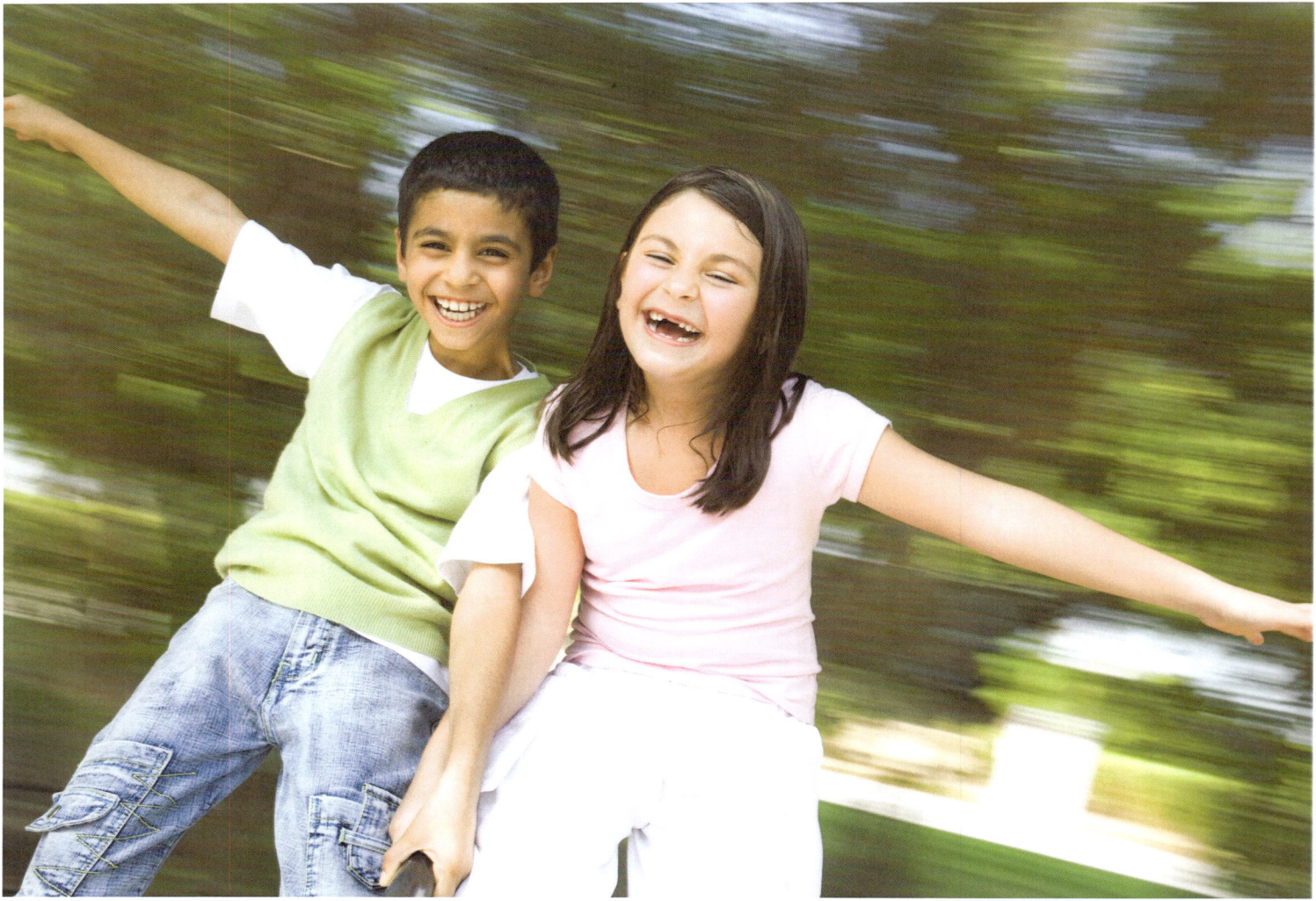

and a happy spirit!

The healthiest foods are lean foods, high in nutrition and low in fat. Lean foods help you feel fit and energized.

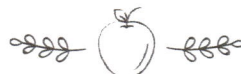

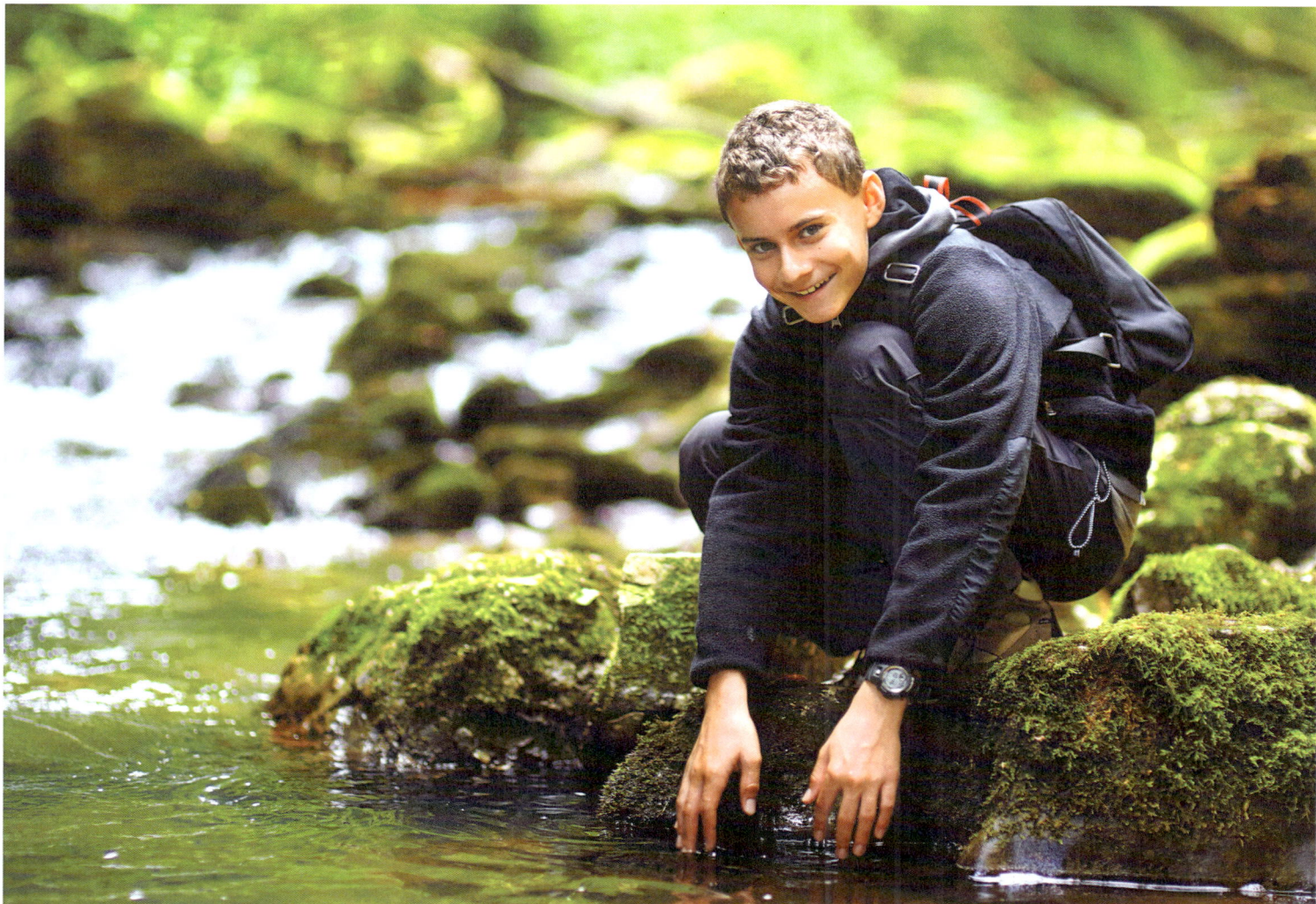

When you choose healthy and lean meals, you'll also be making a difference.

Eating lean helps to keep our planet green, saving precious natural resources like rivers, forests and animals.

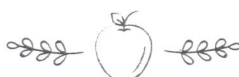

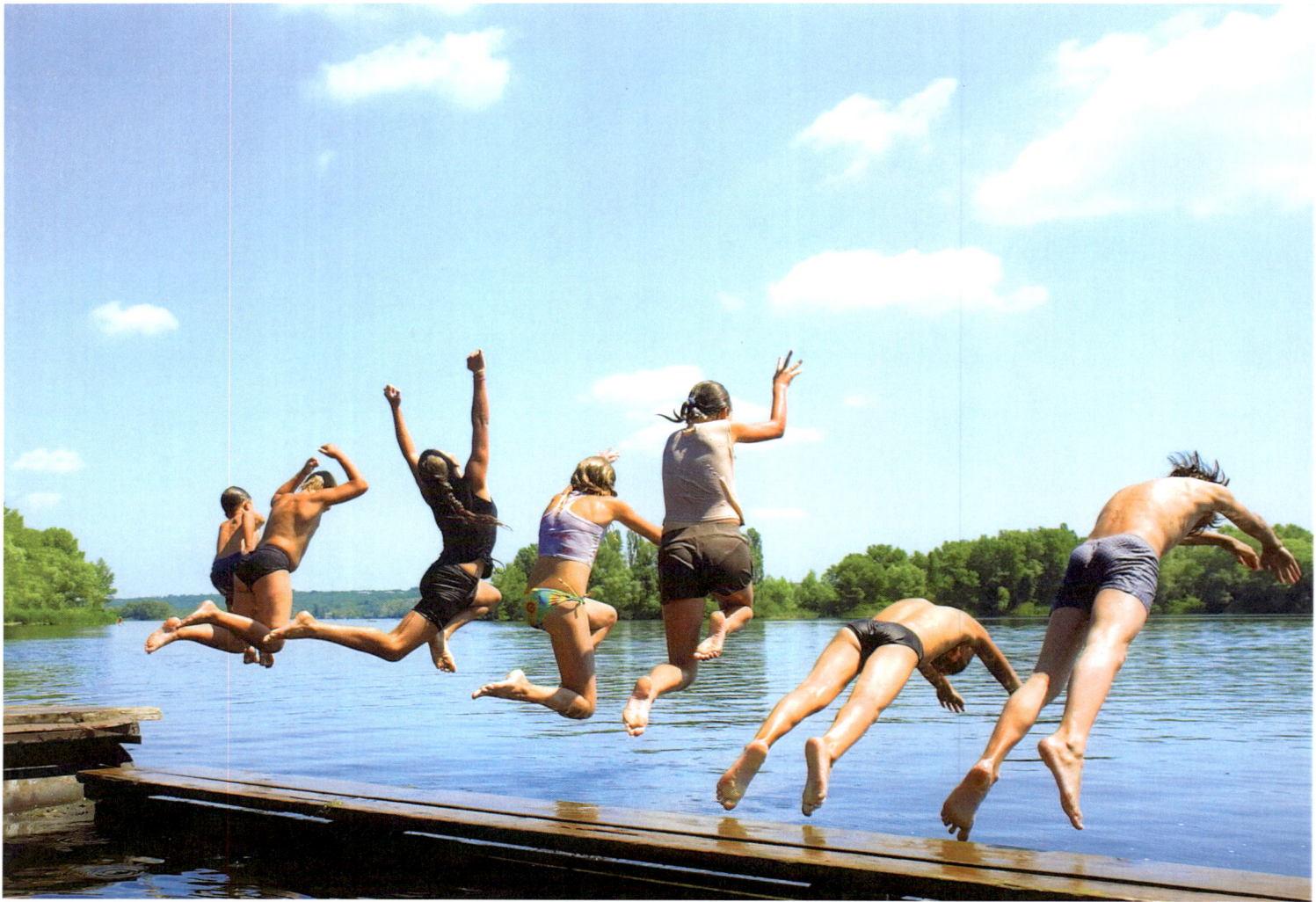

Eating *lean and green* is good for you and the planet too!

Eating *lean and green* is easy, with three simple steps.

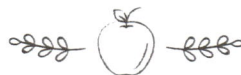

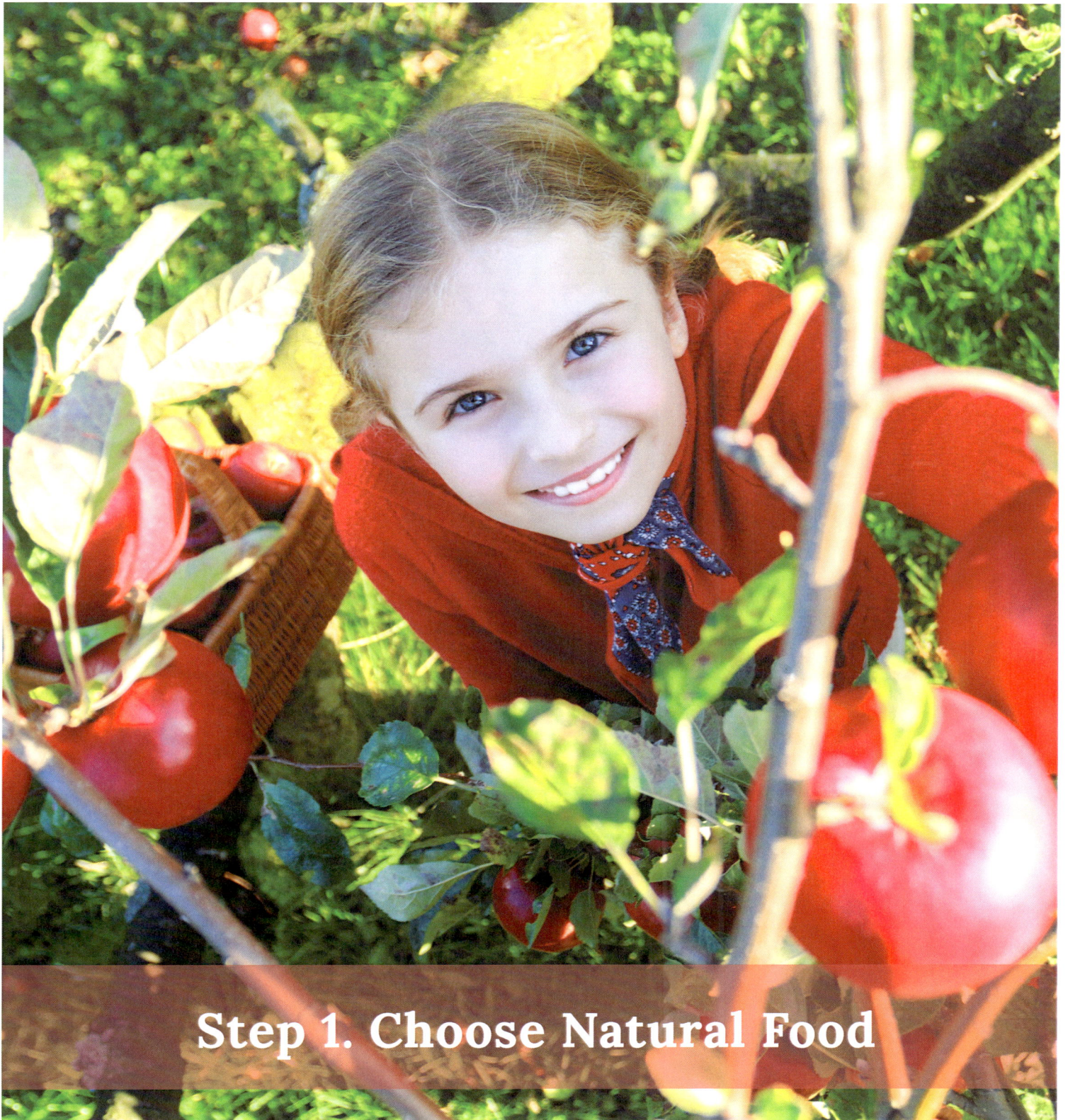

Step 1. Choose Natural Food

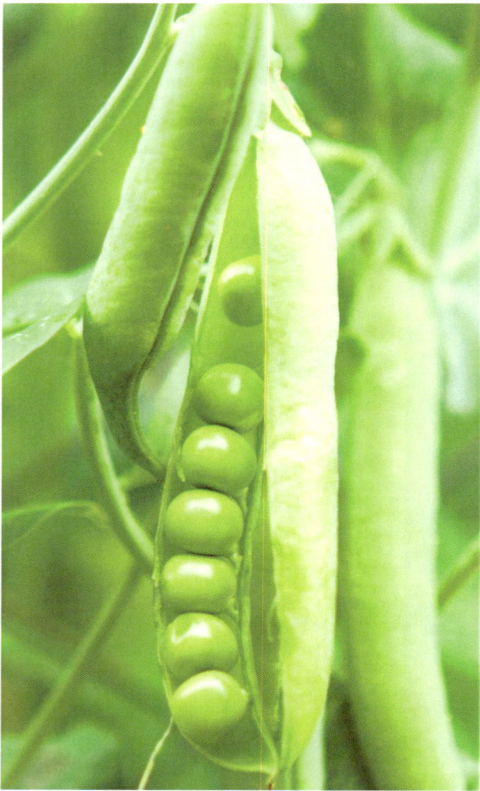

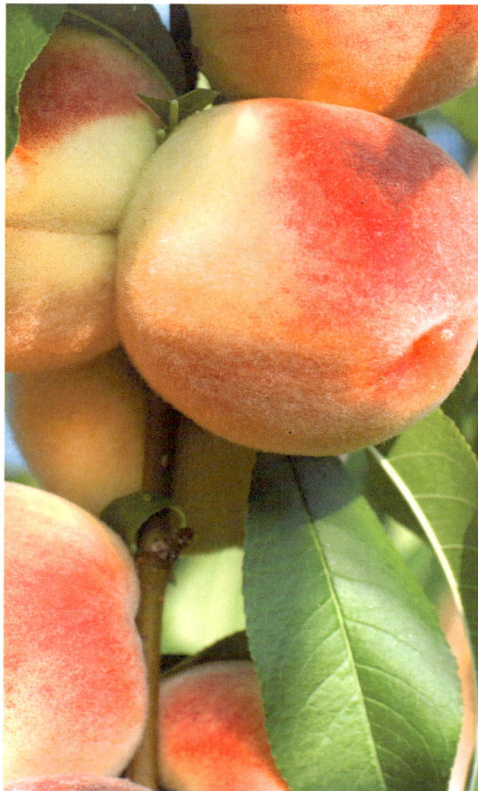

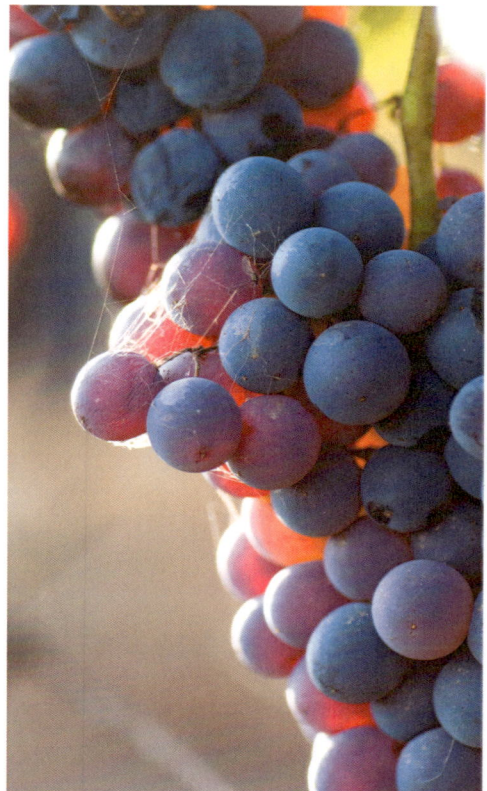

Natural food grows from the earth, like fruits and vegetables.
They're good for you because they're rich in nutrients.
Nutrients are things like vitamins, minerals and protein.

They provide the nourishment you need to live and grow.
The more nutrients you eat, the stronger, smarter and
happier you will feel.

Different colors of food represent different nutrients, which is
why it's important to eat a rainbow of colors everyday.

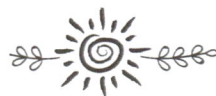

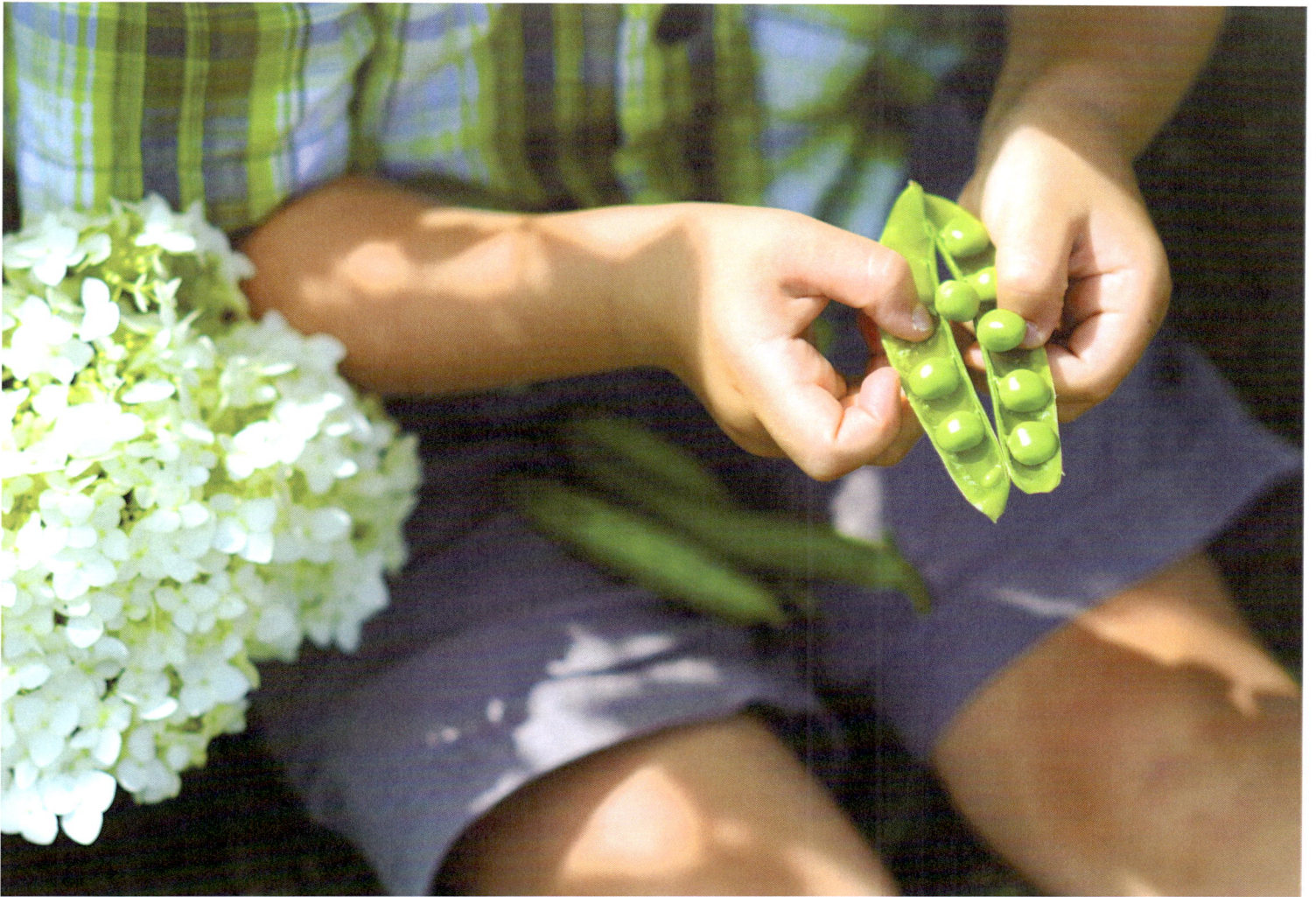

Beans and peas are a special type of vegetable called a legume. They grow in pods. Beans and peas are rich in the nutrient protein. Protein is important for building strong muscles, including your heart muscle that beats 100,000 times a day!

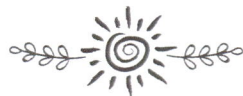

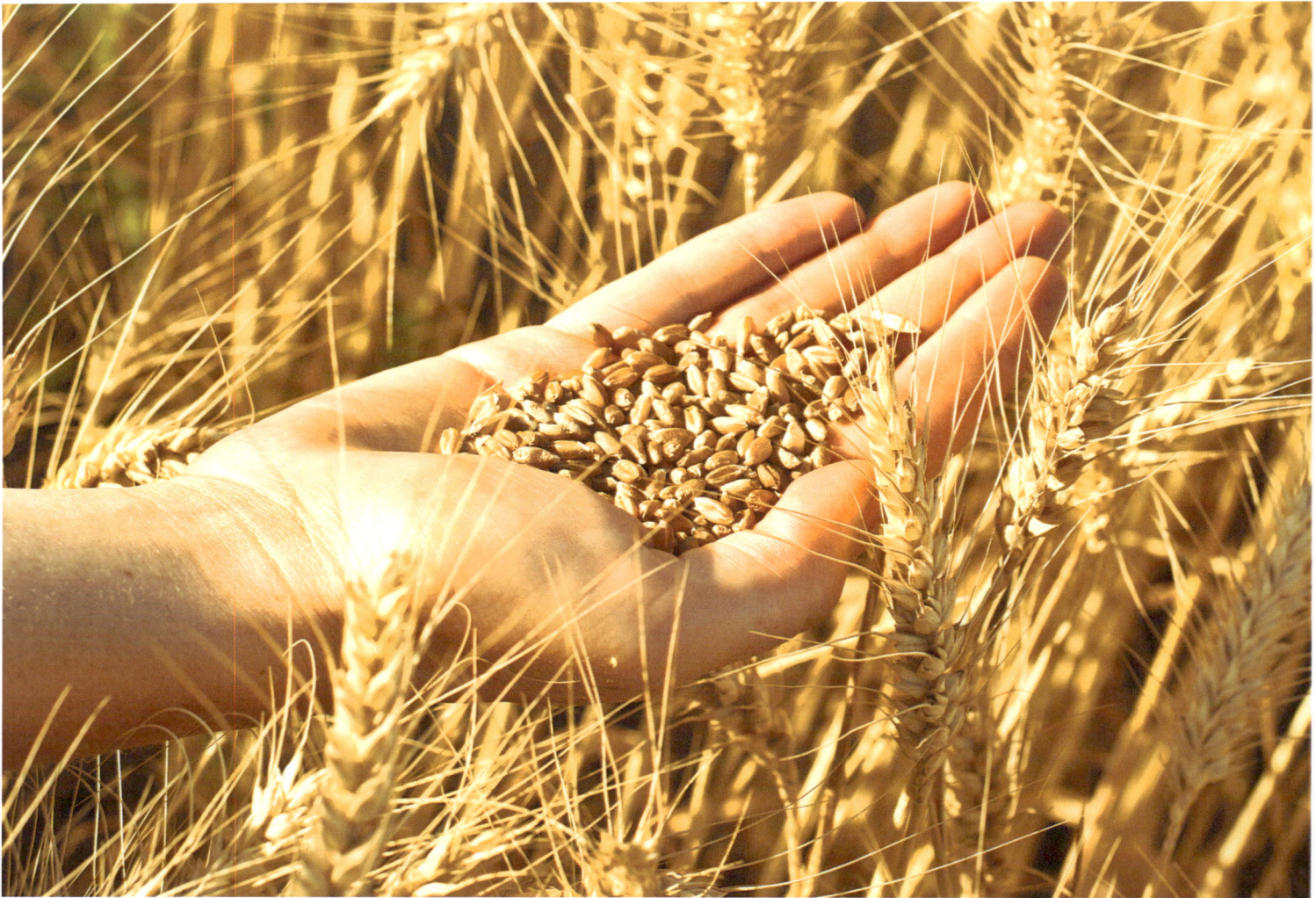

Grains are also natural foods that grow from the earth.
They are the seeds of tall grasses that once grew wild.

Oats are grains for making oatmeal.
Wheat is a grain to make bread.

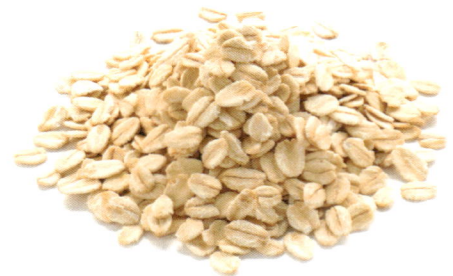

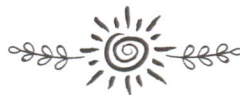

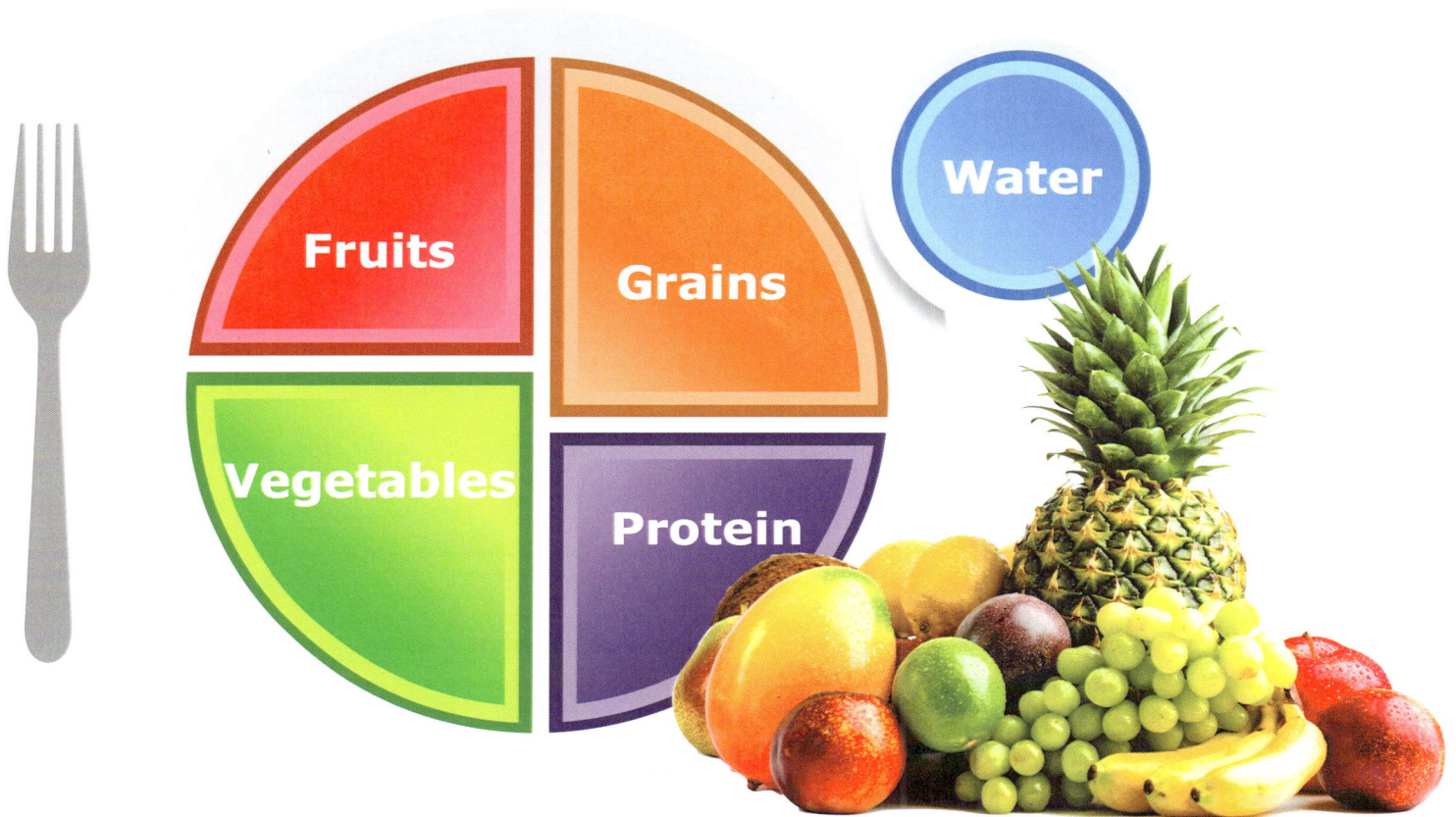

*Harvard School of Public Health, *Healthy Eating Plate.*

The Healthy Eating Plate* is a good model for eating *lean and green.* Fruits, vegetables, grains and protein-foods are all natural and healthy foods. They grow from the earth, pure and simple.

Plants are one kind of natural food. Can you guess the other?

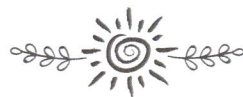

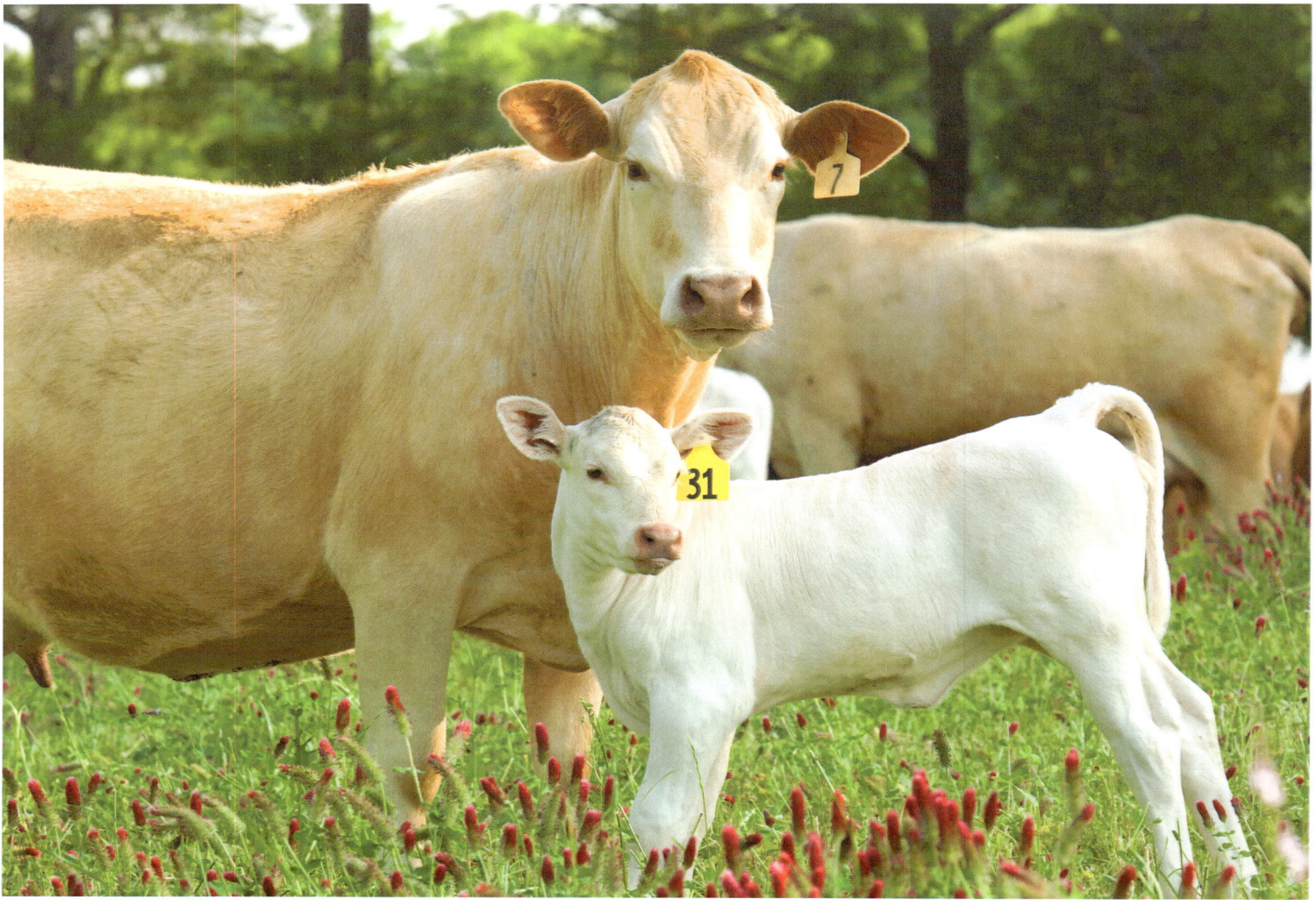

Animals are the other natural food. They are part of Earth's natural ecosystem. Steak and hamburger meat are made from cows.

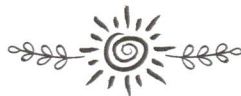

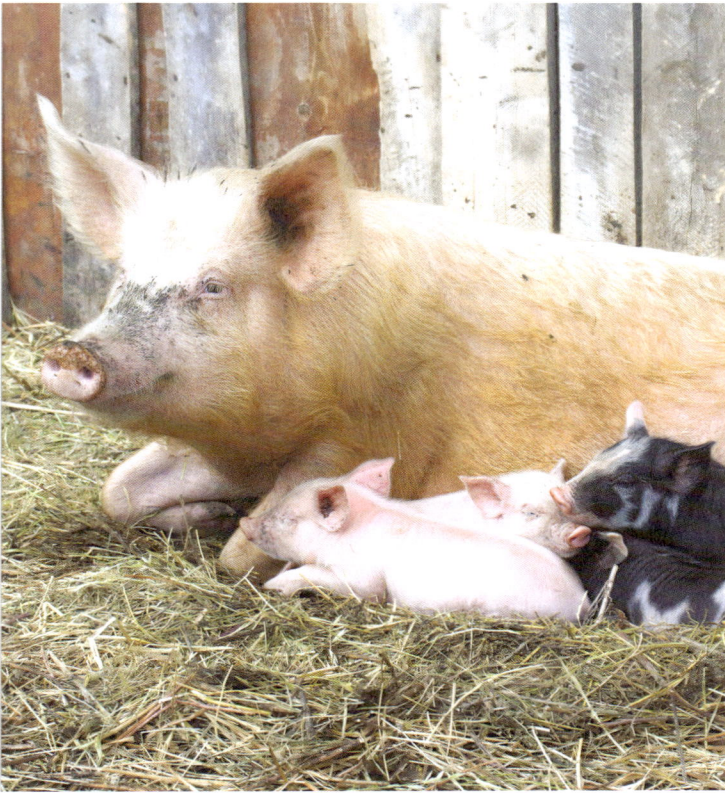

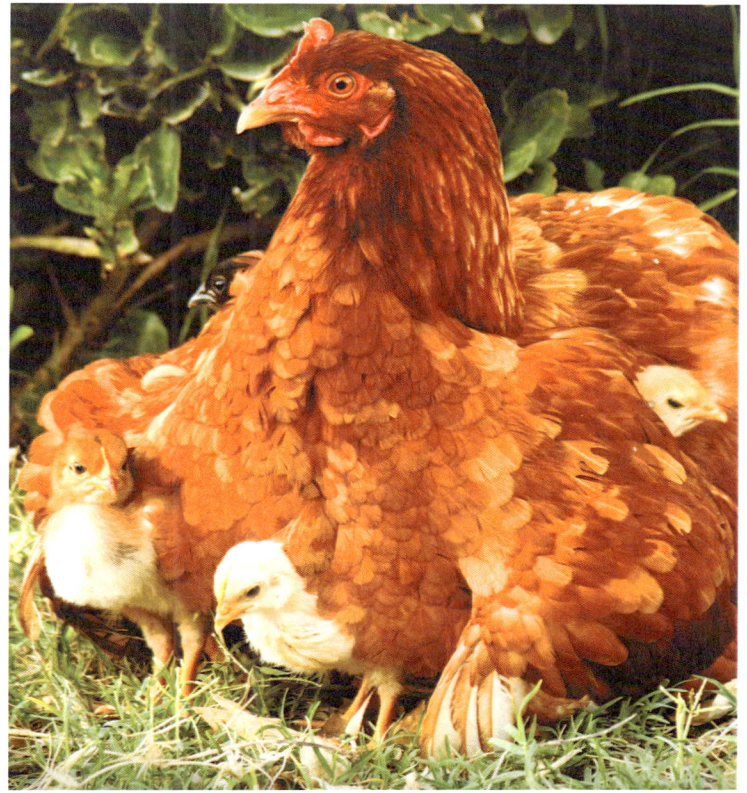

Ham and bacon are made from pigs. Chicken nuggets and drumsticks are made from chickens. Animal foods are high in protein. Around the world, people eat animals you might not ever consider eating.

People even eat bugs for protein!

But there are also many people around the world who choose to *not* eat animal food at all. A person can get all the protein they need from plant foods, like grains and beans.

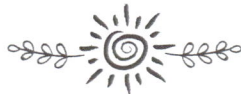

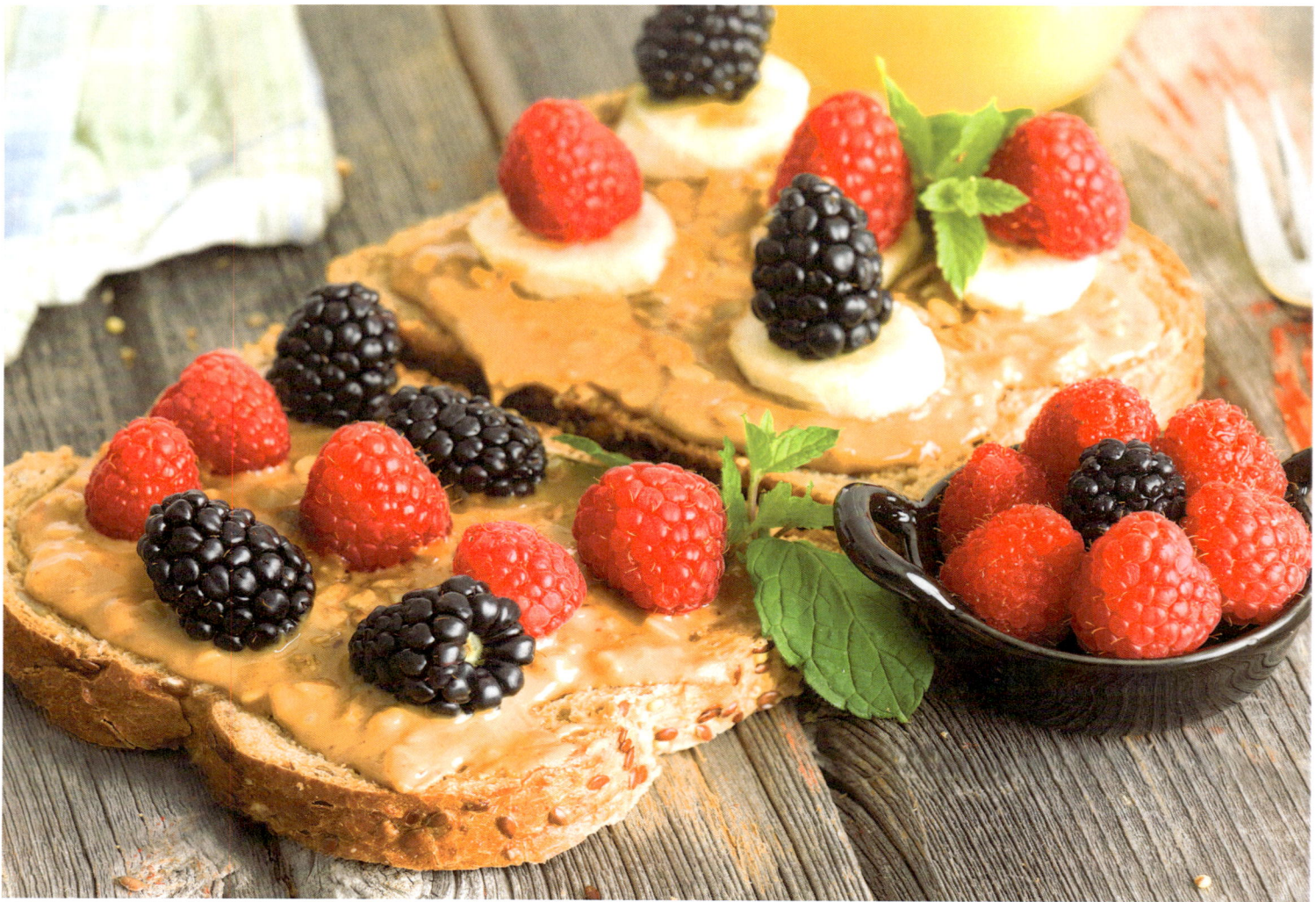

So, natural food comes from plants and it comes from animals. That's all. The opposite of natural foods are processed foods, sometimes called "junk food."

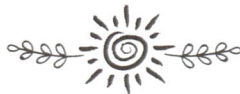

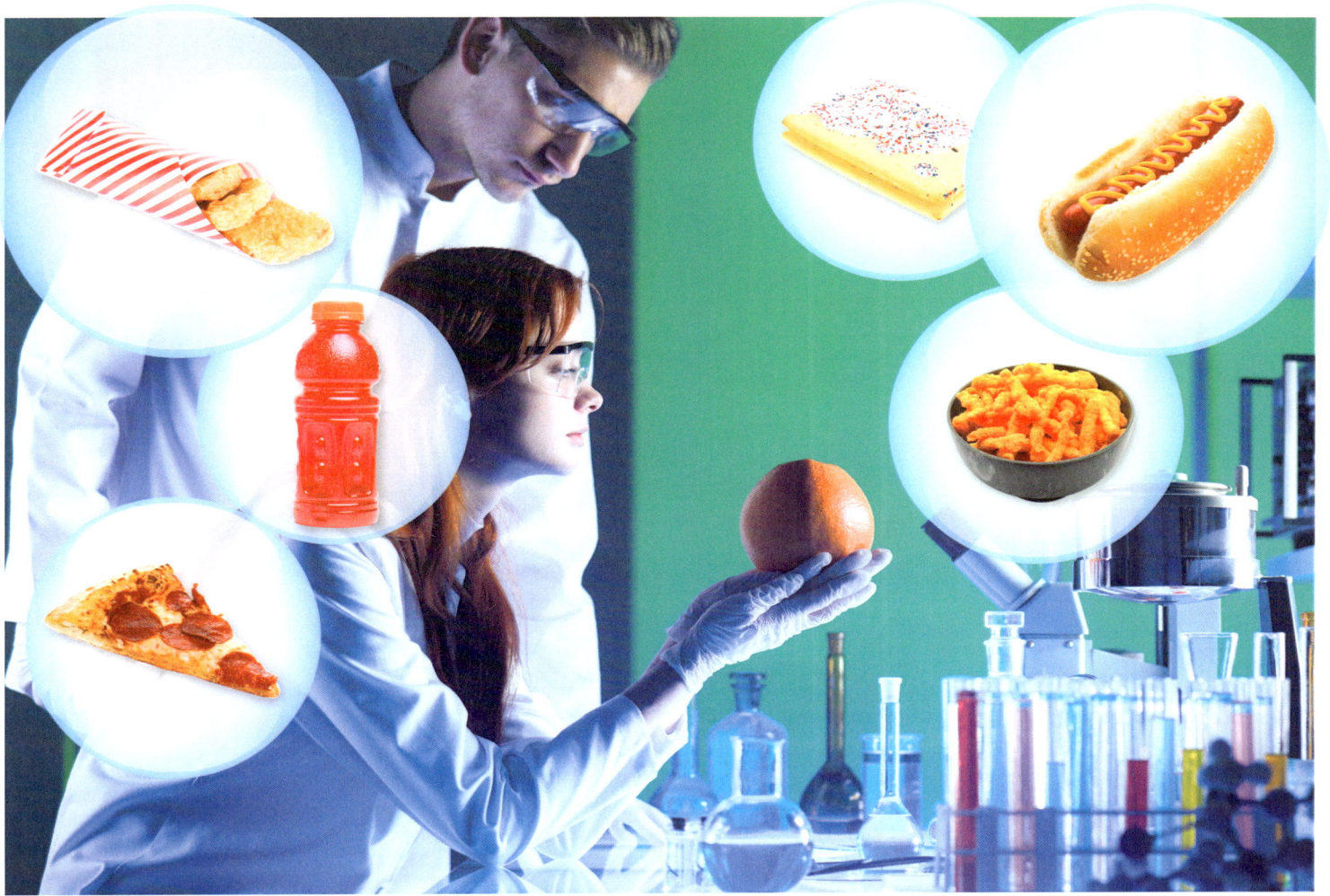

Processed foods are created when big food companies add unhealthy and unnatural ingredients to make their products more tempting.

Processed foods are low in nutrients and can leave you feeling tired and grumpy.

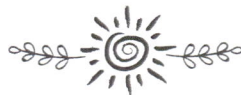

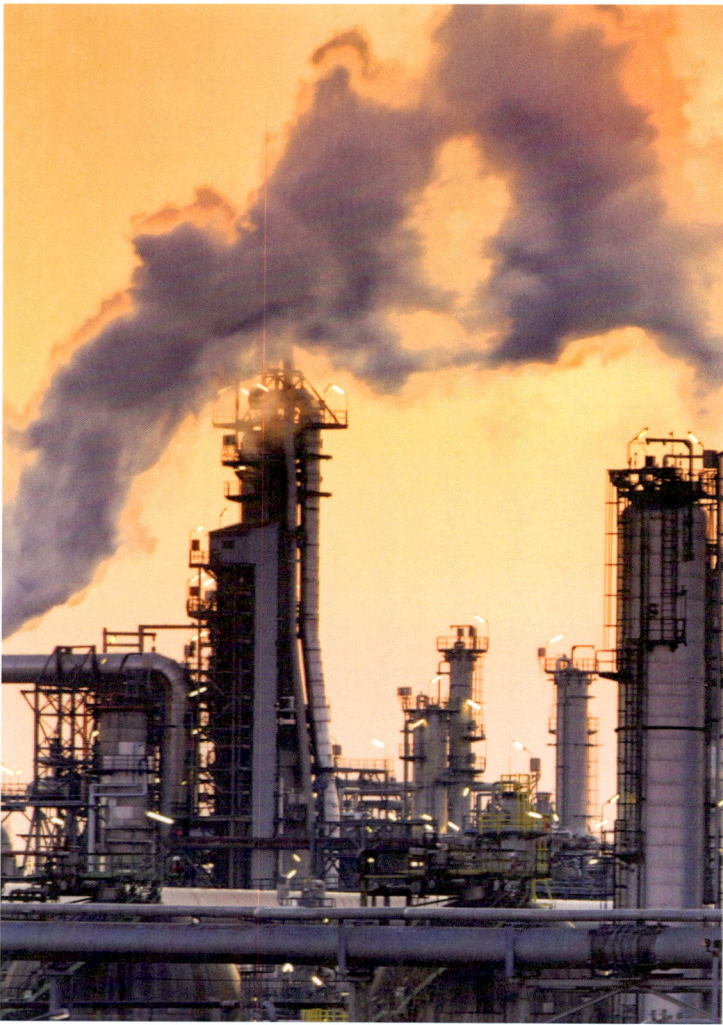

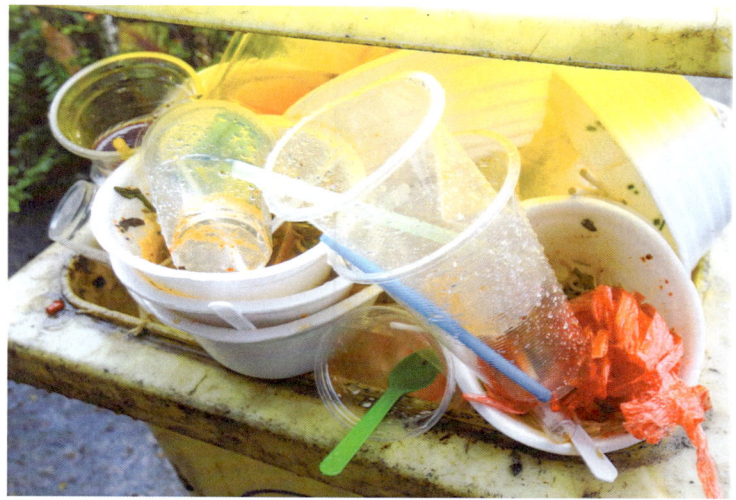

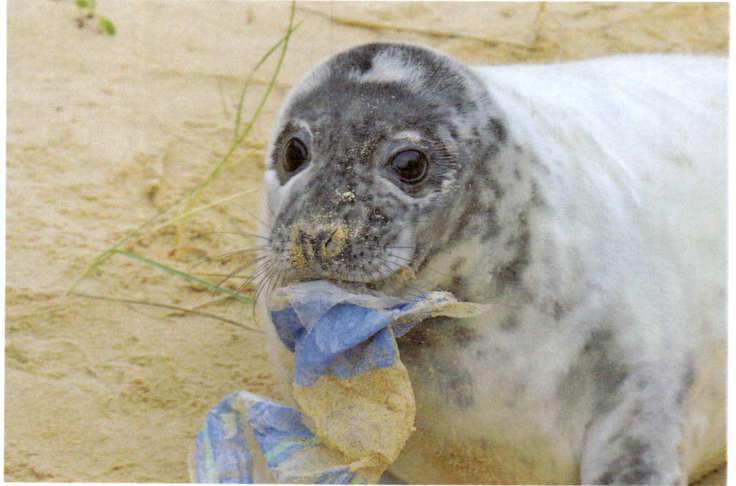

Processed foods are not *lean and green* choices.

Processed foods can harm your body and the planet.

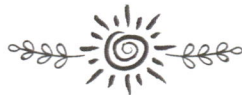

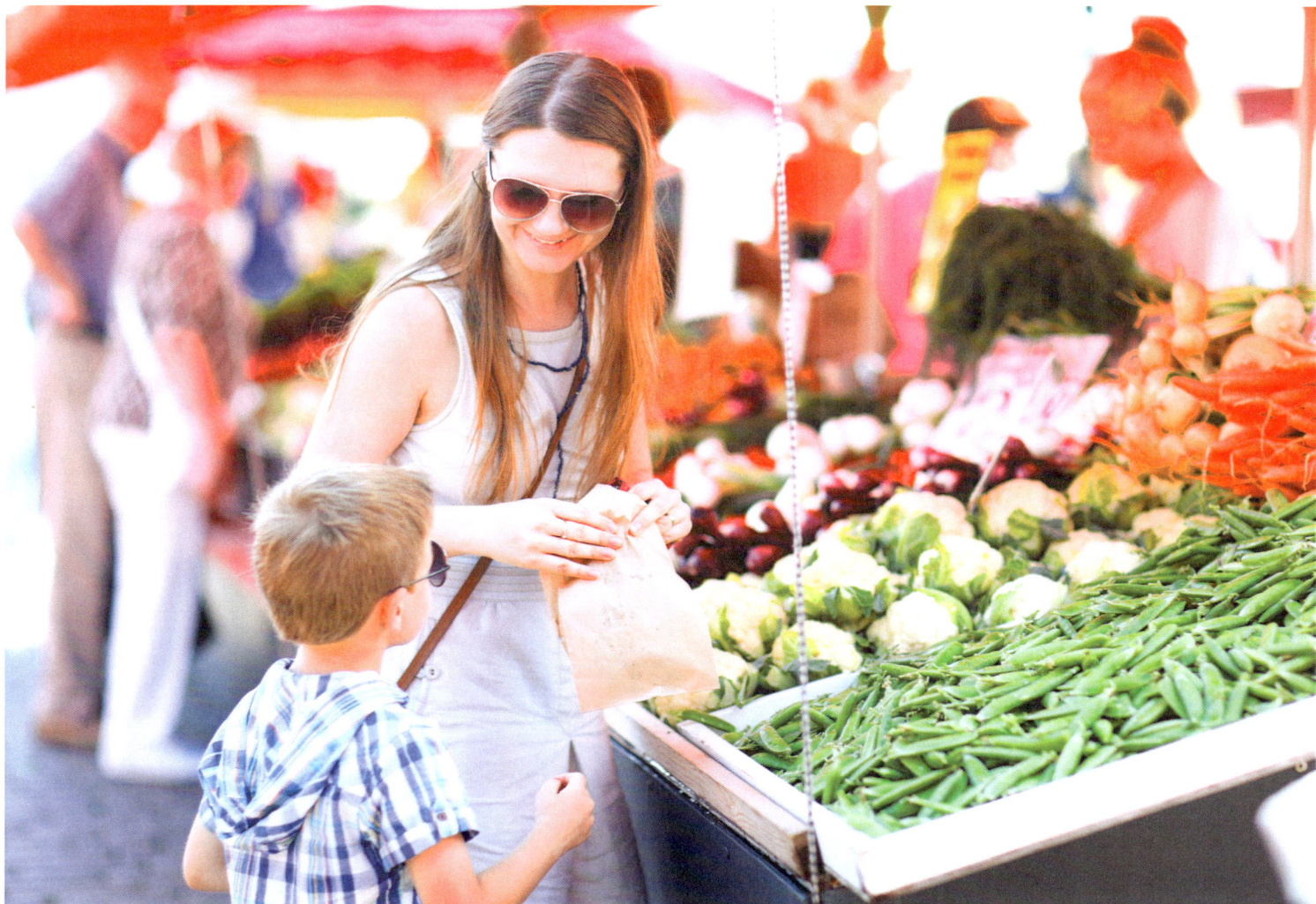

Natural foods are not created by big food companies and produced in factories. They're grown by farmers, farmers you can meet at your local Farmer's Market.

Wherever you shop for food, remember that when you choose natural food, you have taken the first important step for eating *lean and green*.

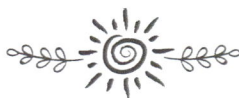

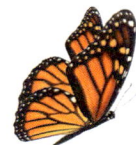

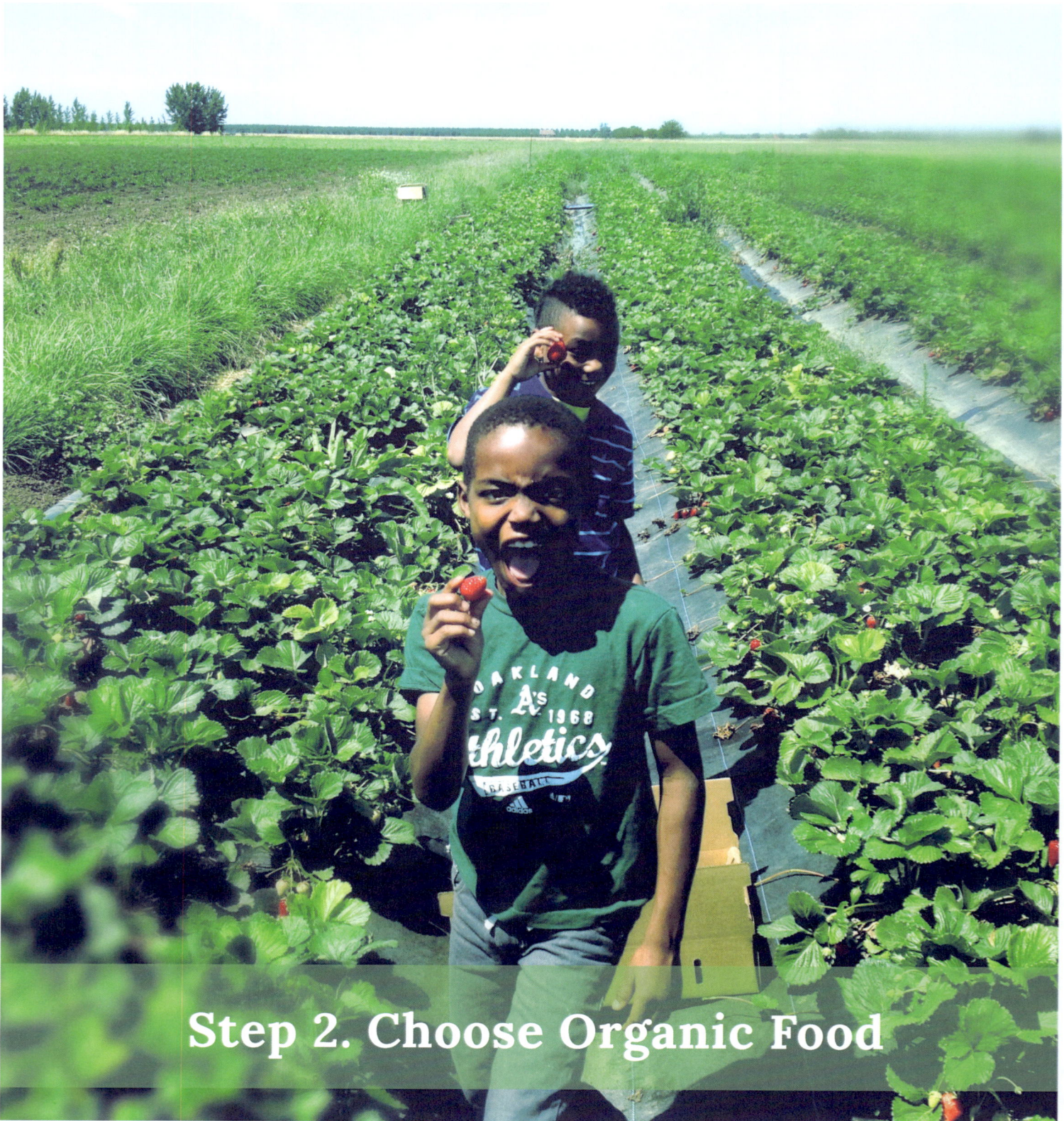

Step 2. Choose Organic Food

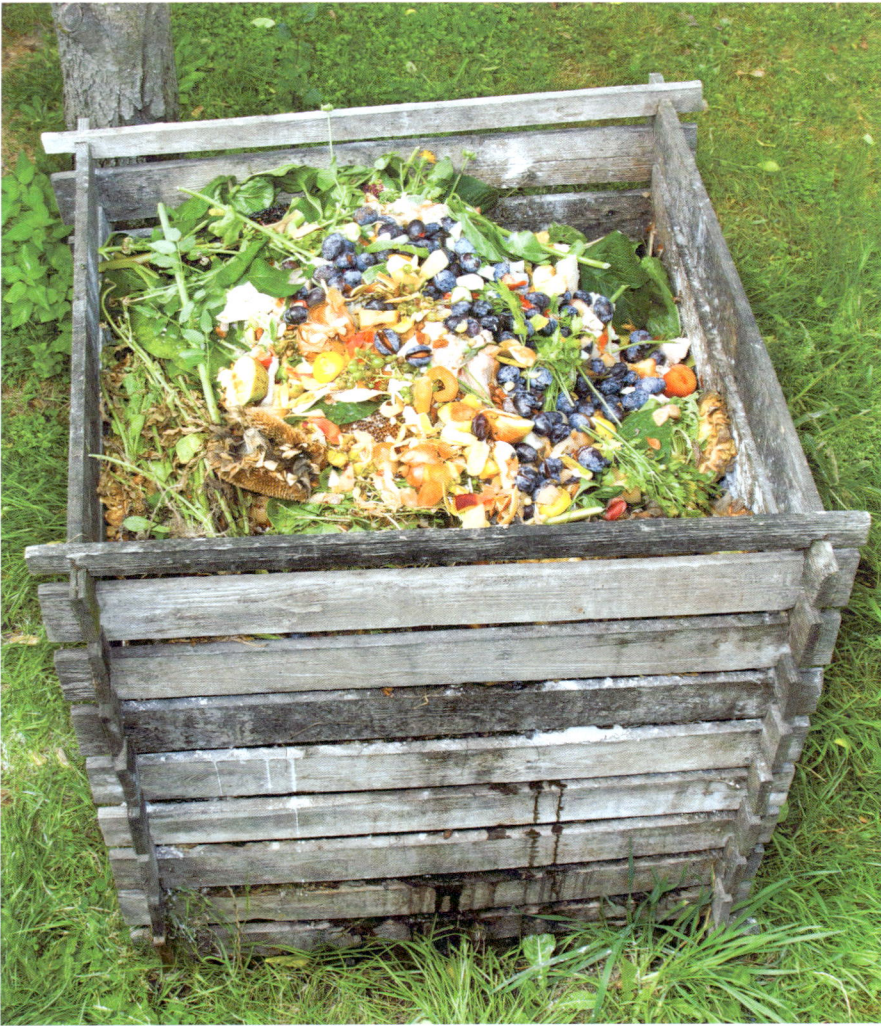

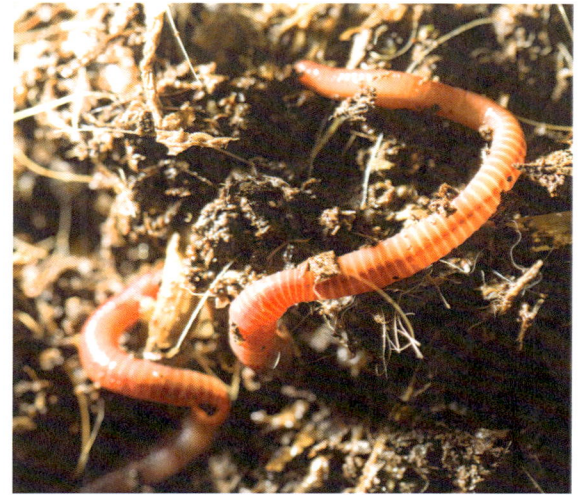

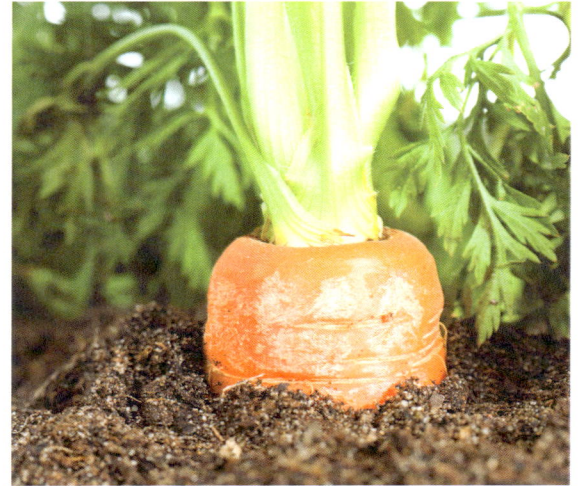

Organic food is grown the old fashioned way, in harmony with nature.

Instead of using man-made chemical fertilizers that can harm the teeny-tiny creatures that live in the soil, organic farmers use natural fertilizer, called compost. Compost is made from dead plants and rotting food! All that dead and rotten stuff actually nourishes the soil and little microorganisms that live in the soil, for growing healthier food and a healthier you!

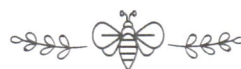

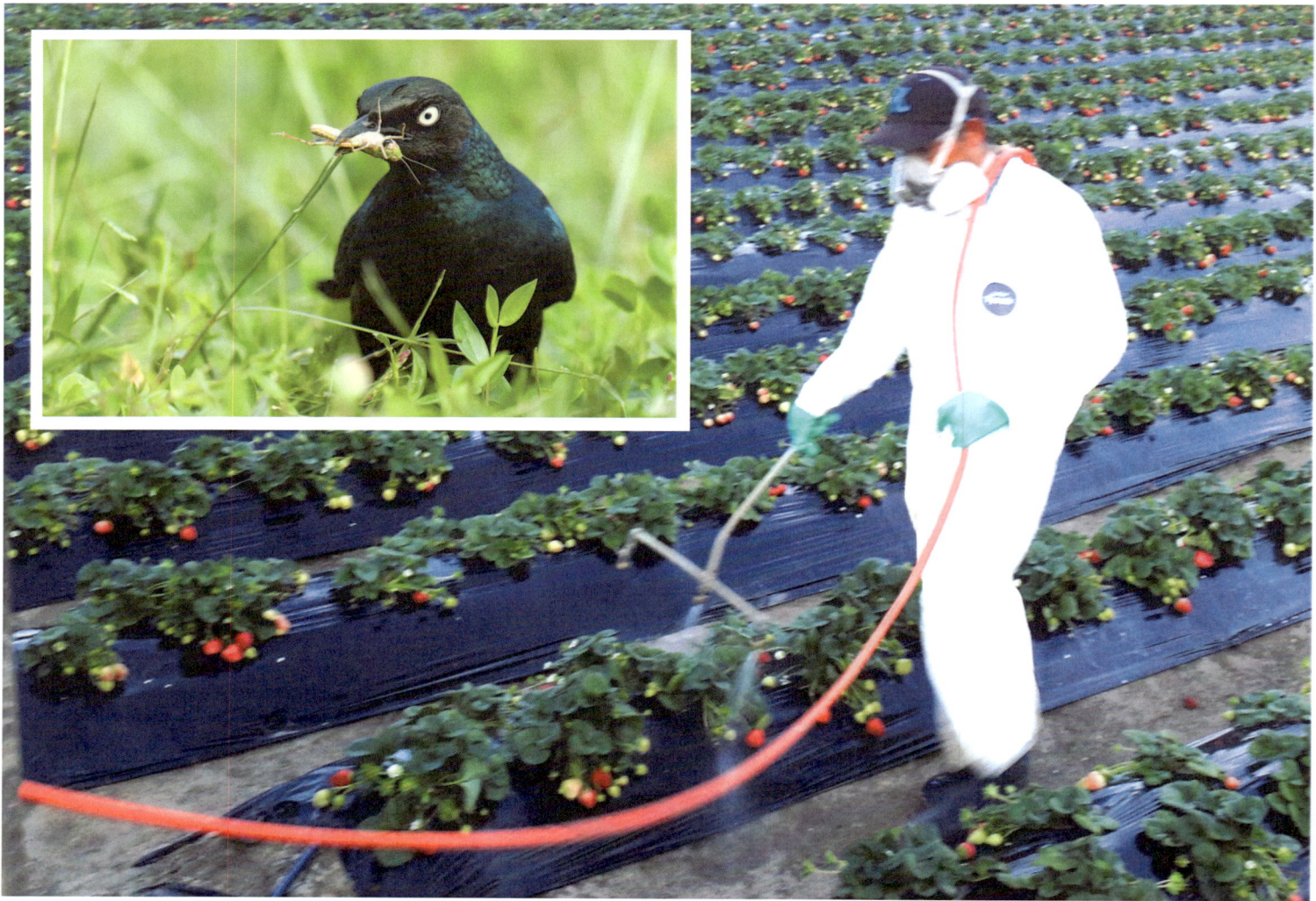

Organic food is also grown without chemical bug poison.
Scientists have discovered bug poison kills beneficial
insects, like bees and butterflies.

It can even kill the birds that eat the bugs that were sprayed.

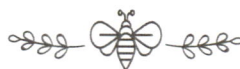

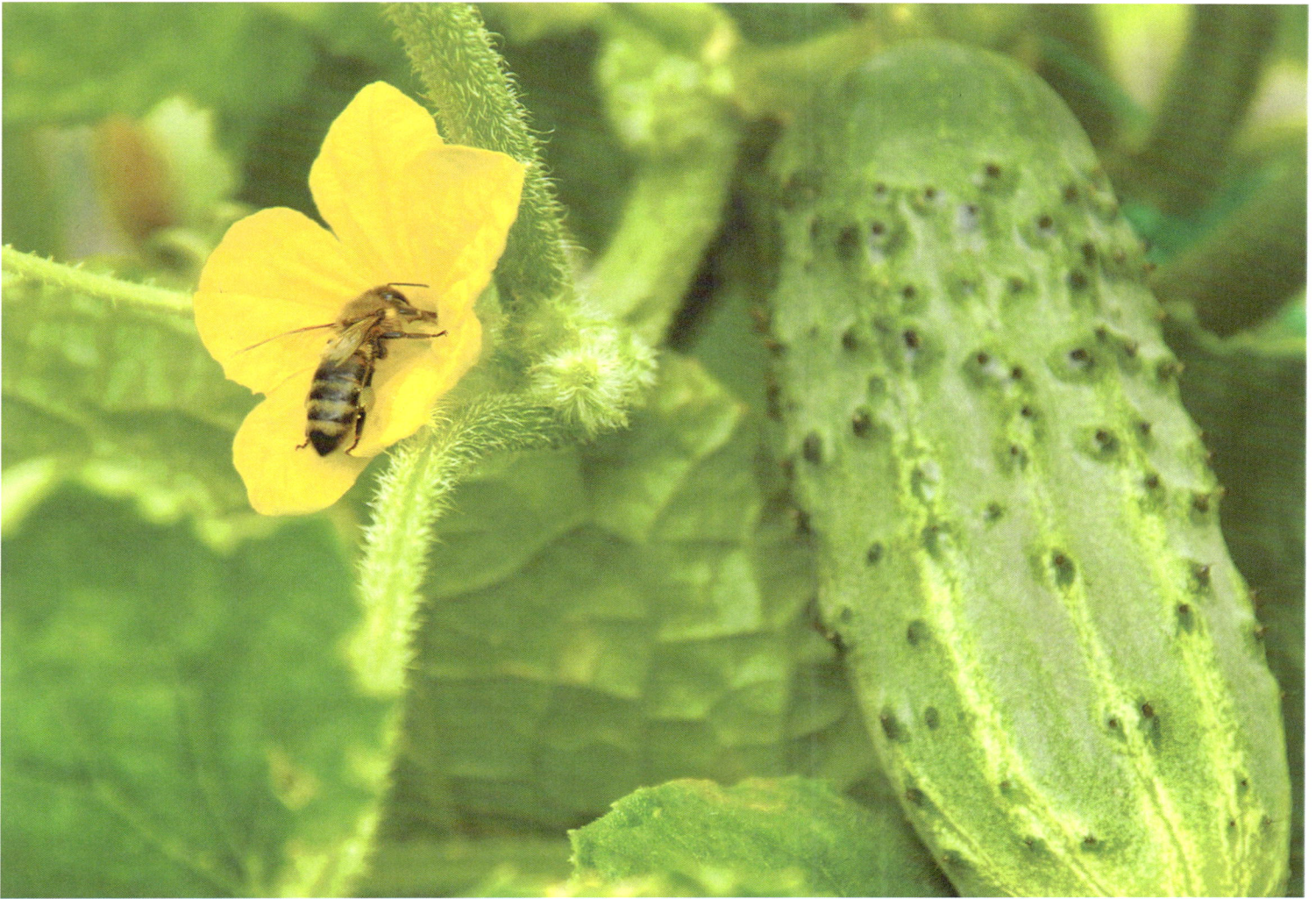

Choosing organically grown food is eating *lean and green*.
It's more nutritious for you and safer for the birds, bees,
and fish that swim in the sea!

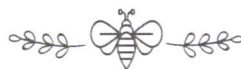

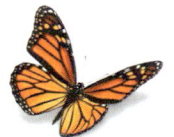

Fruits

Grains

Vegetables

Protein

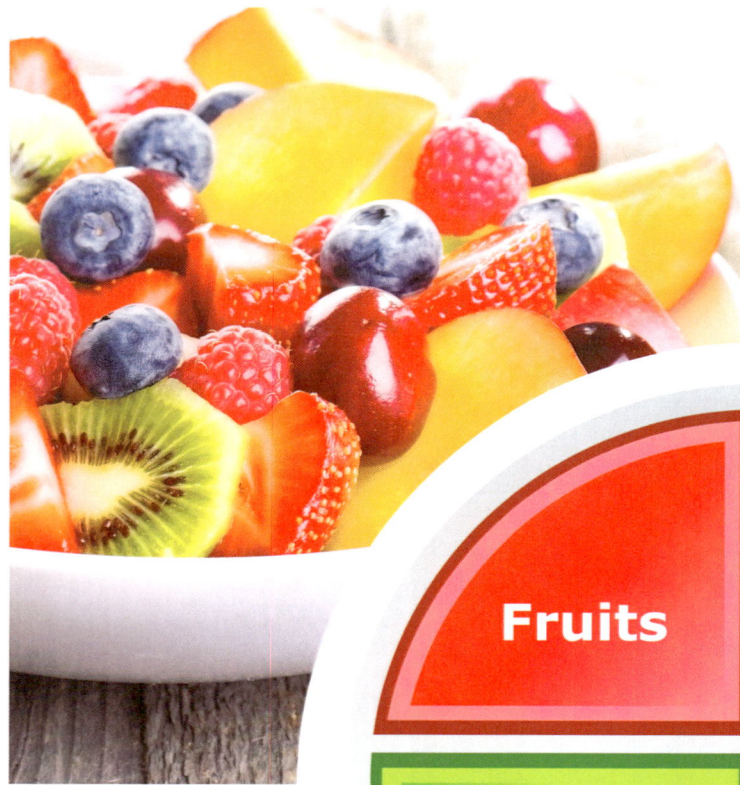

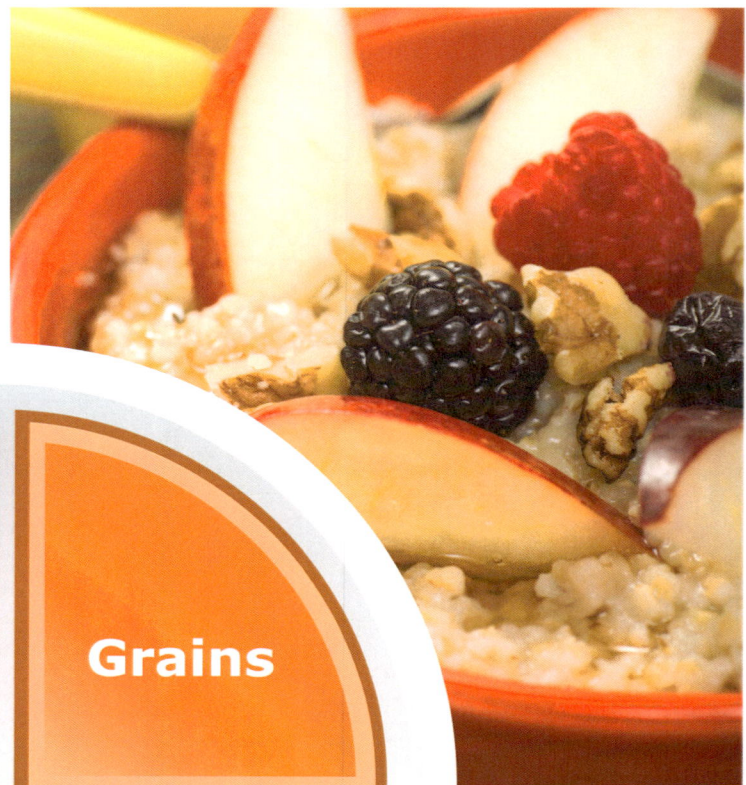

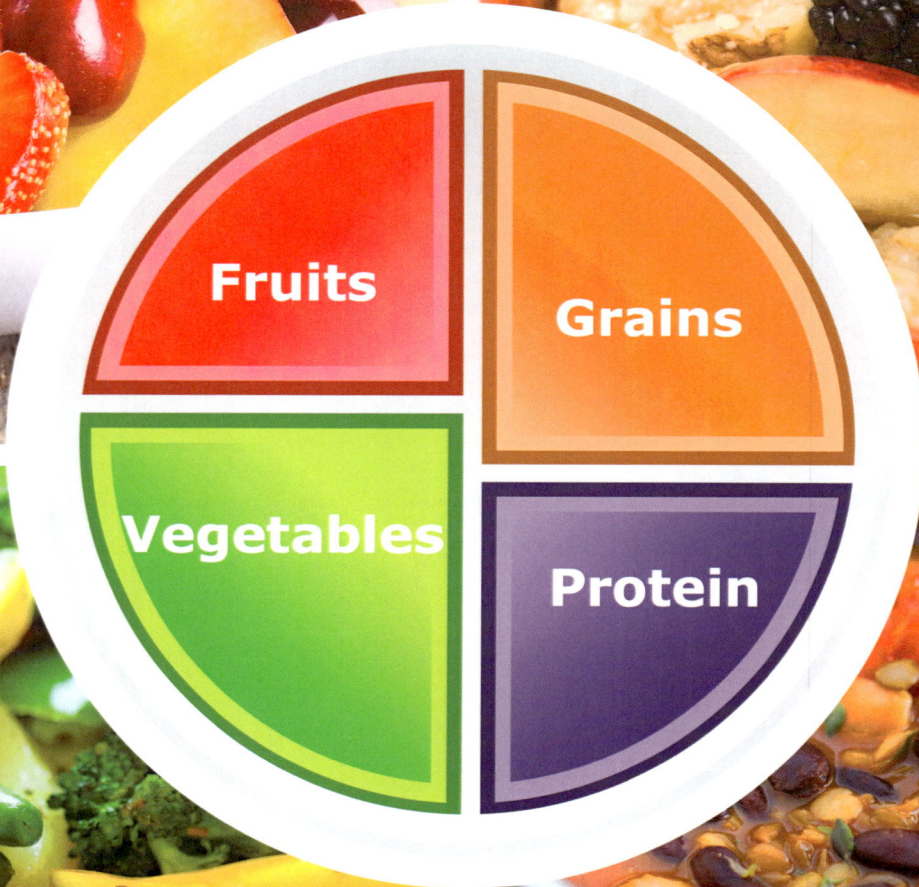

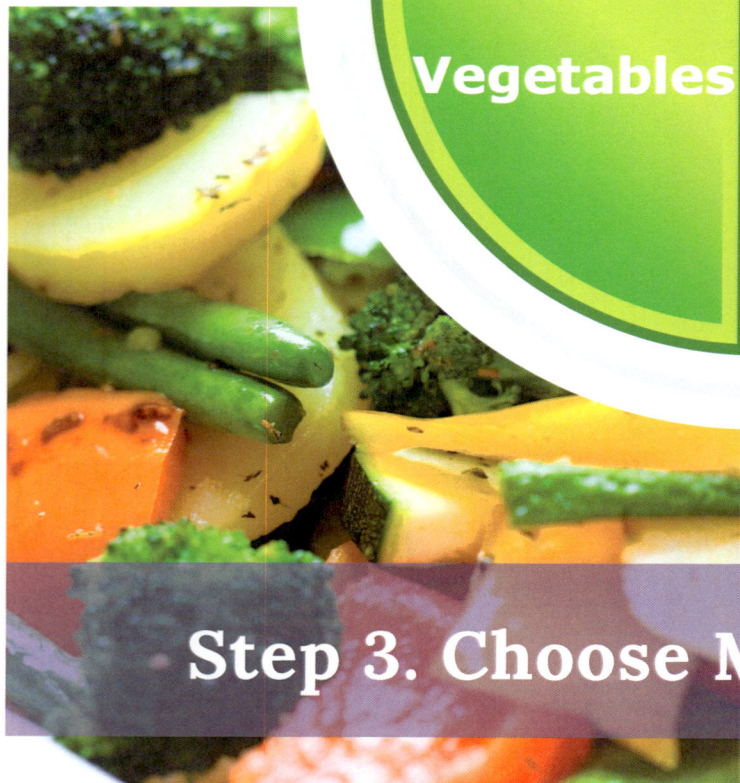

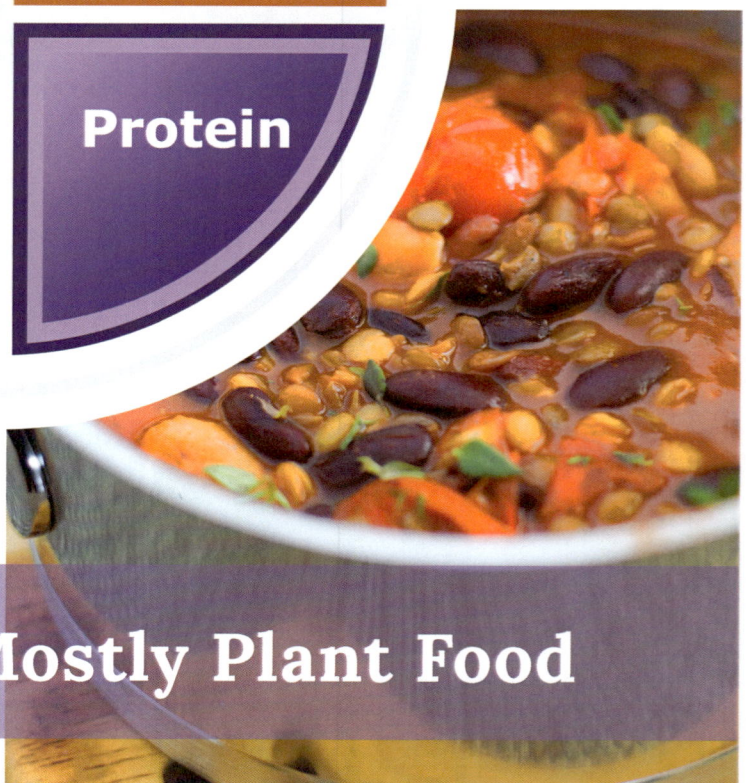

Step 3. Choose Mostly Plant Food

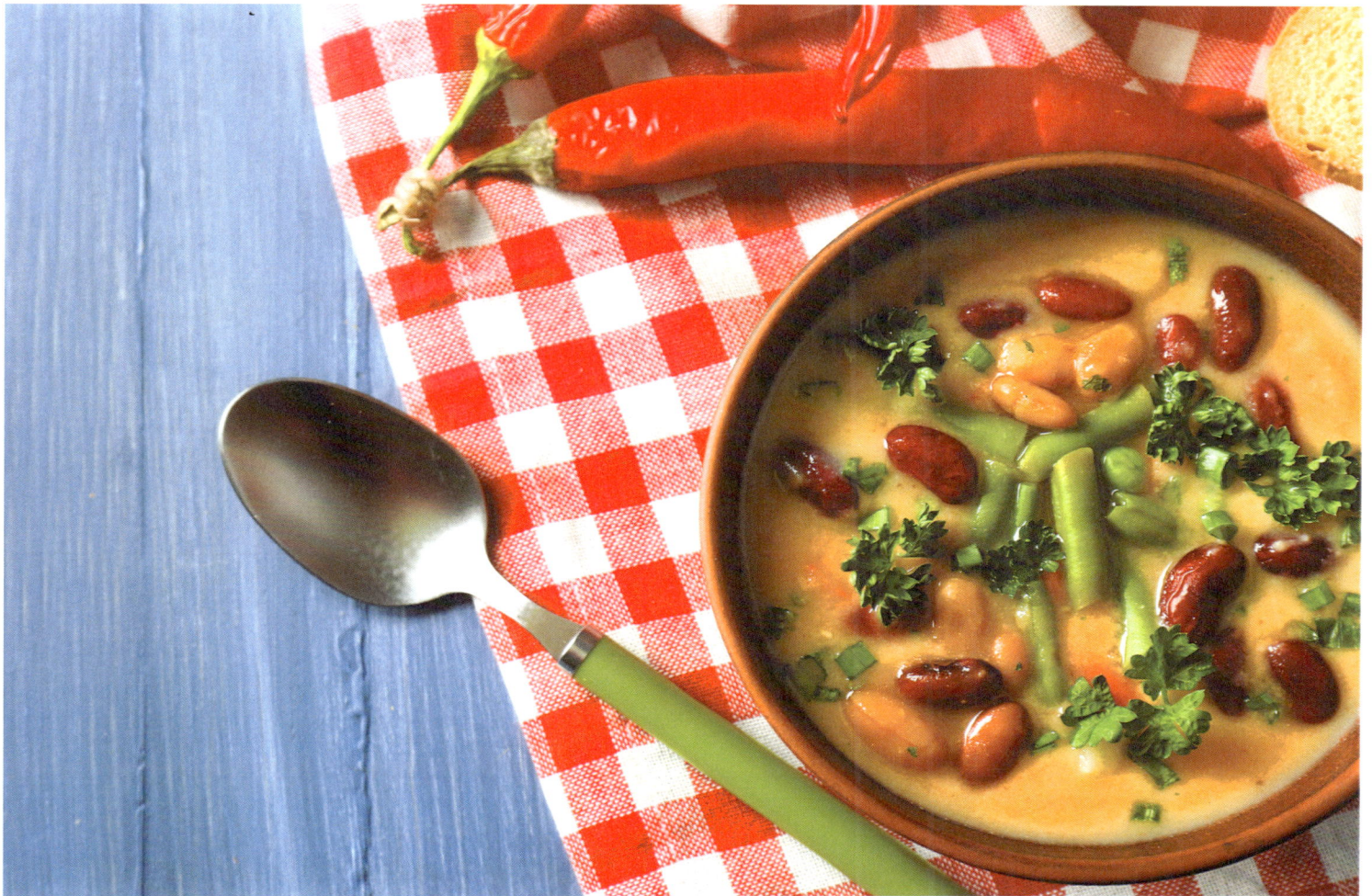

Plant foods have up to ten times more nutrition than animal foods! And only plant foods have super special nutrients called *phytonutrients*. Like the name suggests, phytonutrients help fight disease for a longer and stronger life.

Beans are the lean and green protein choice. They are a plant-protein. Here's a fun fact: Scientists studied people around the world who lived the longest, and discovered... they all ate mostly beans for protein!

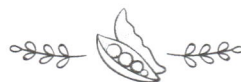

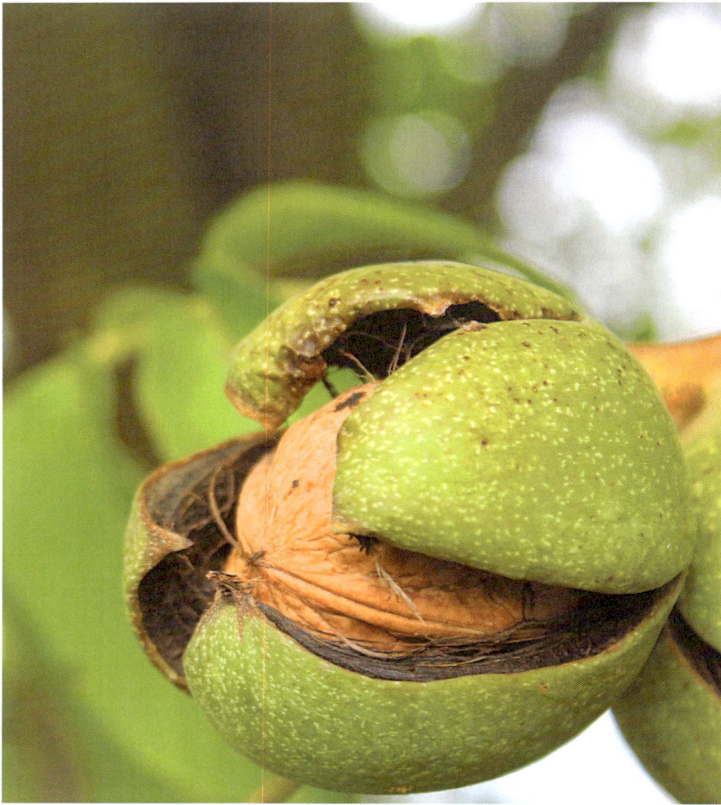

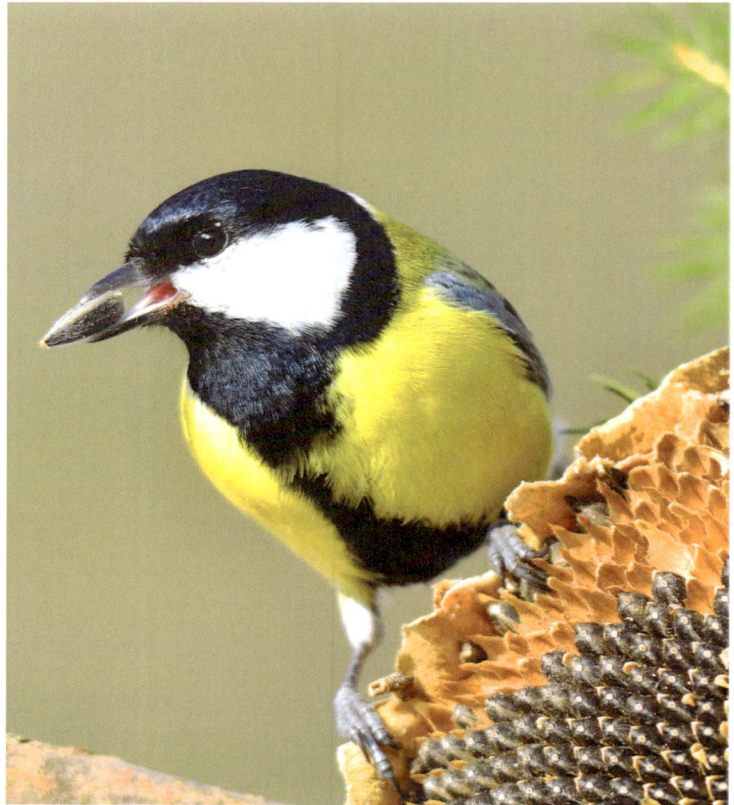

Nuts and seeds are the other *lean and green* plant-protein, with super special phytonutrients to fight disease.

Nuts and seeds boost your brain power too, for tackling those tricky math problems and brainstorming brilliant sentences.

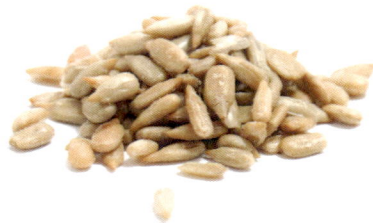

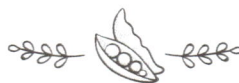

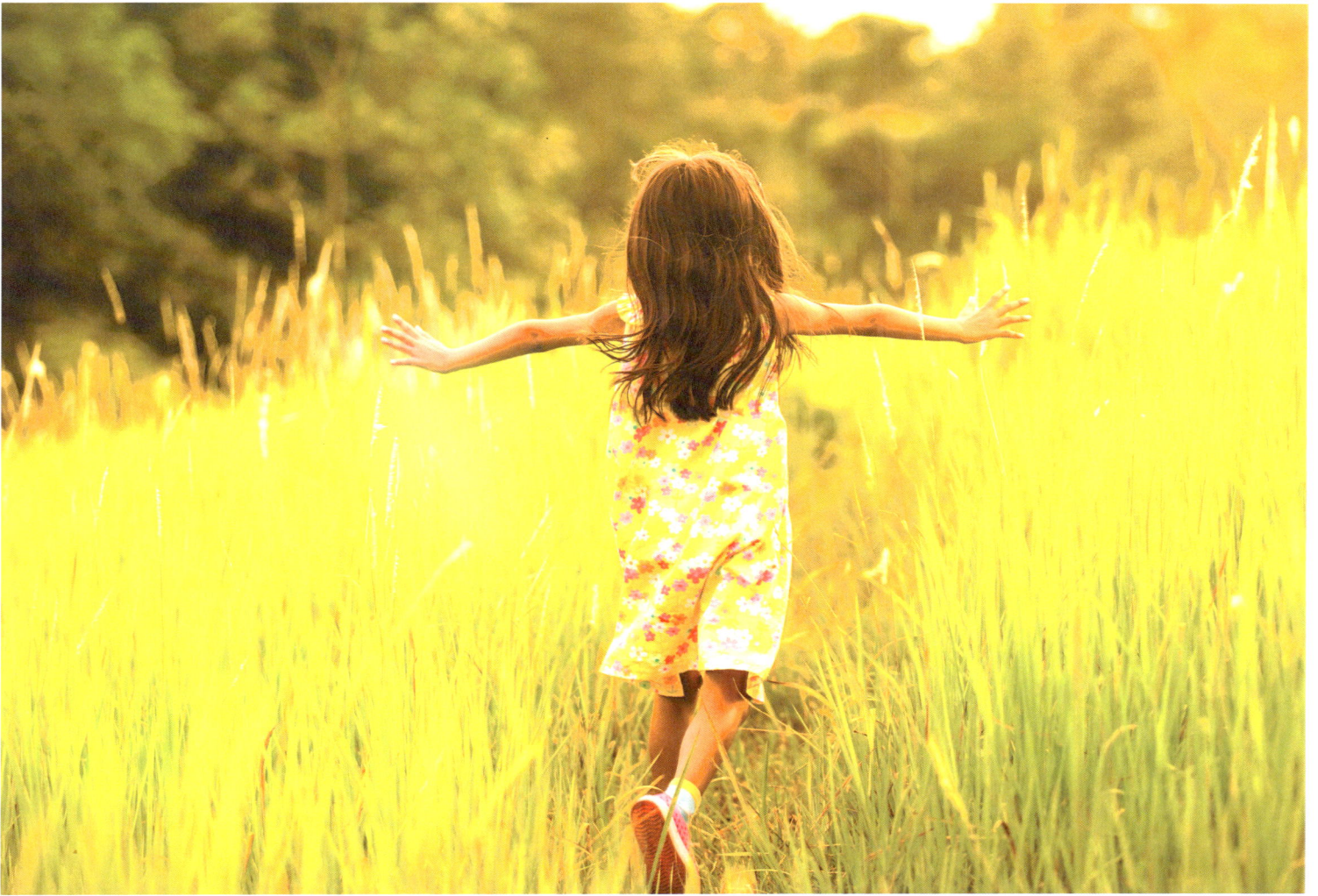

Plant foods are the foundation for growing up strong, smart

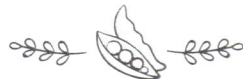

and

happy!

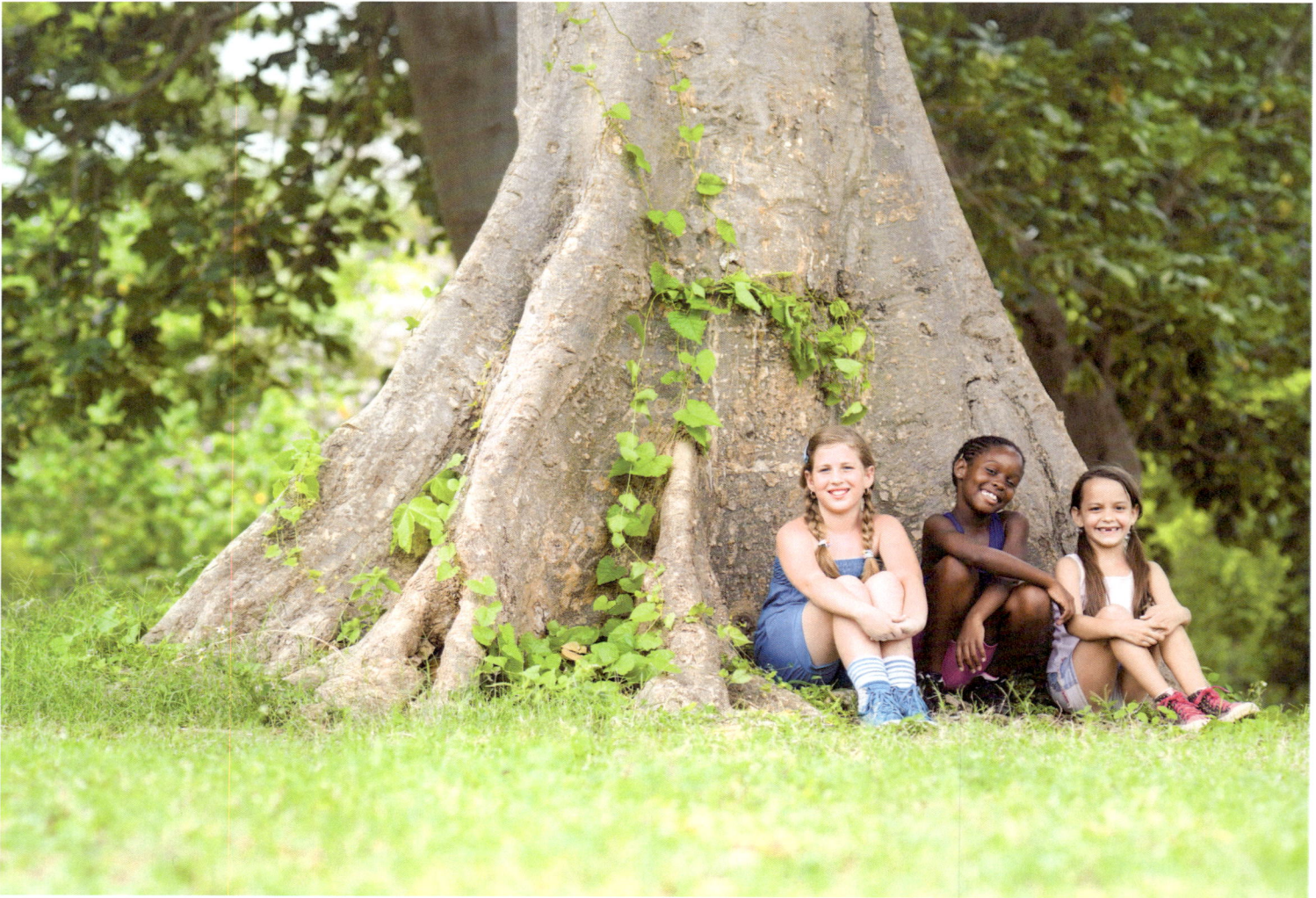

And by choosing plant-based meals, you will be making a difference for the planet too. Raising animals for protein uses up massive amounts of Earth's precious natural resources.

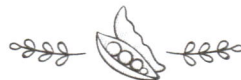

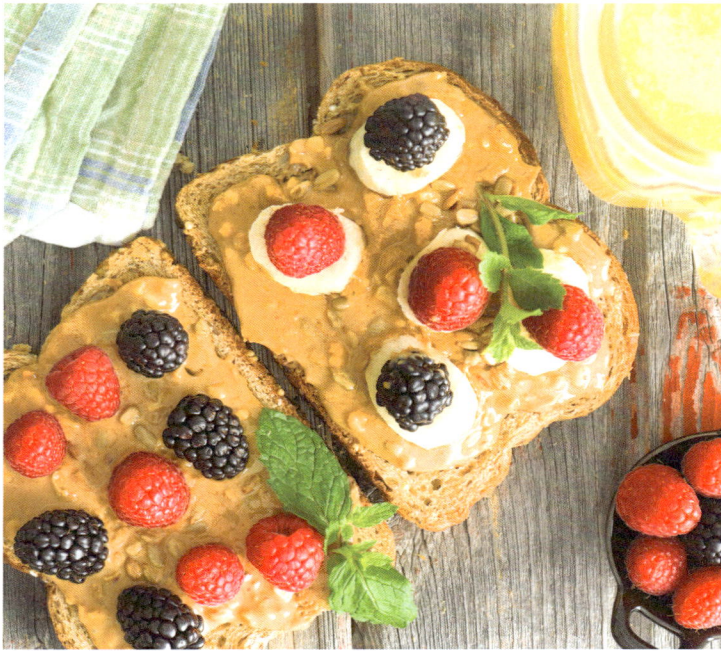
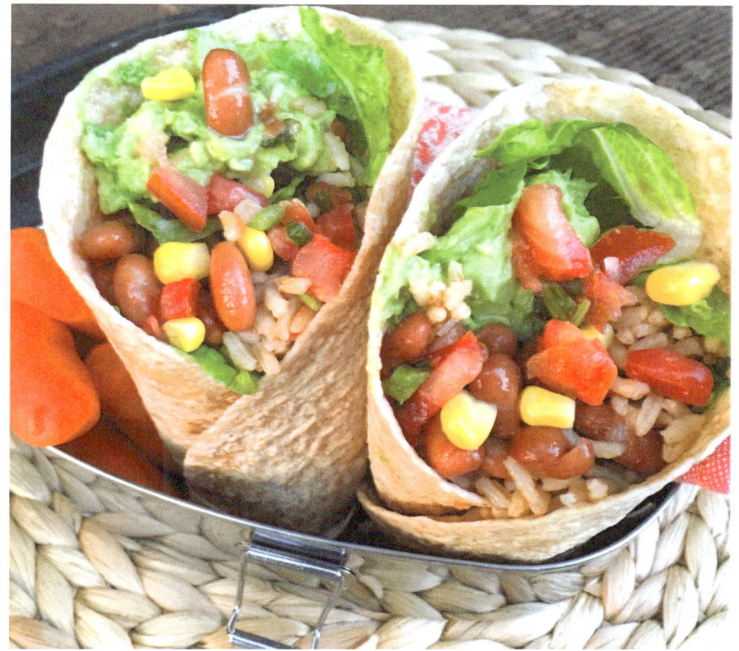

Choosing just one plant-powered meal with nuts or beans for protein conserves over a 100 gallons of water and enough land to grow 100 trees! But there's more.

When you choose a good old peanut butter and jelly sandwich instead of a ham and cheese sandwich, or a bean burrito instead of a beef burrito, you'll help conserve as much energy as turning off all the lights in your house for a whole month!

Conserving energy helps cool our planet and reduce global warming.

Cool Beans!

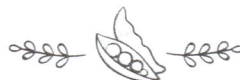

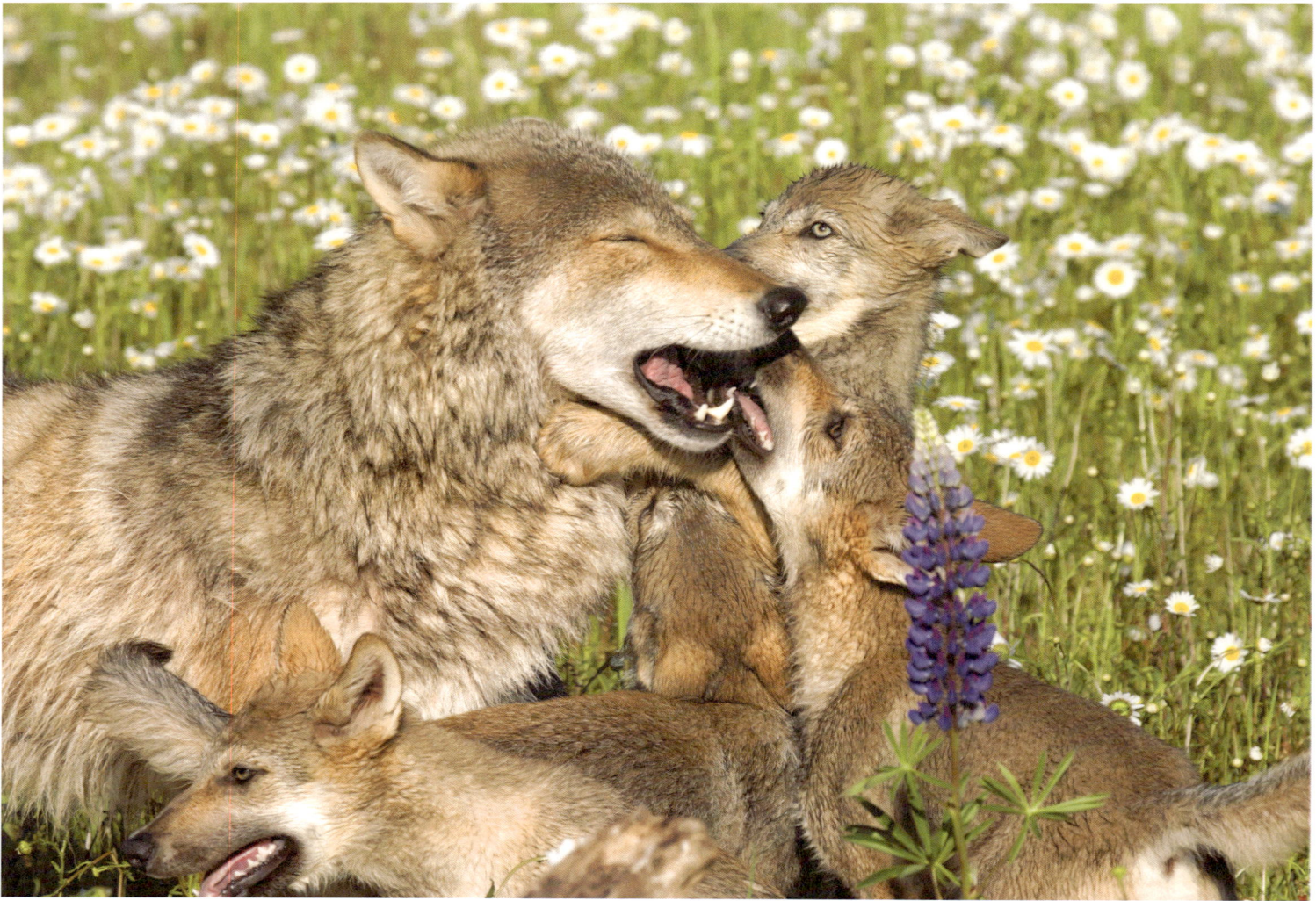

Saving water, land and energy all help to save wild places and wild animals too.

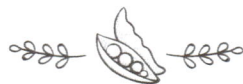

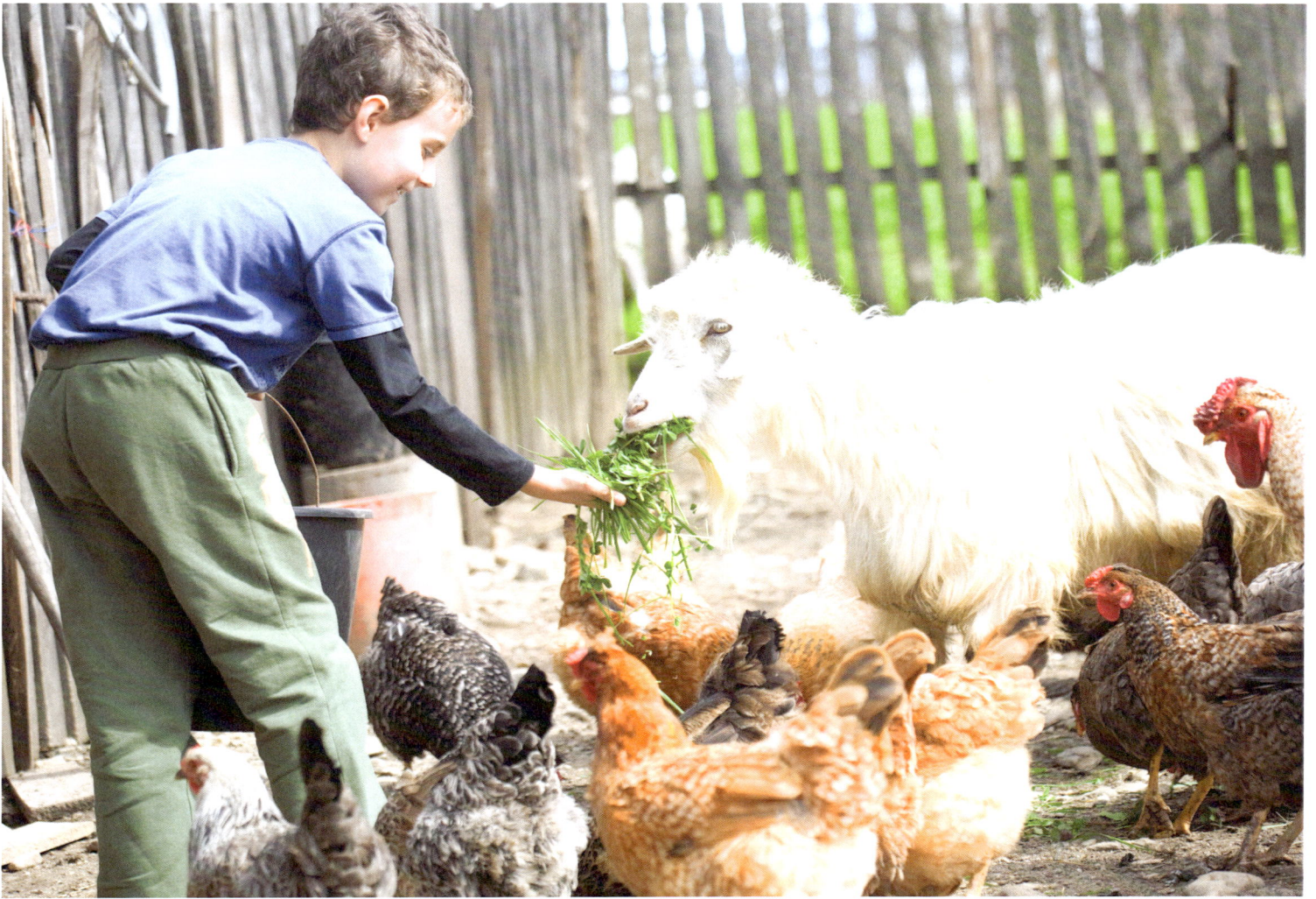

Plant-based meals also help farm animals.

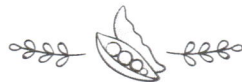

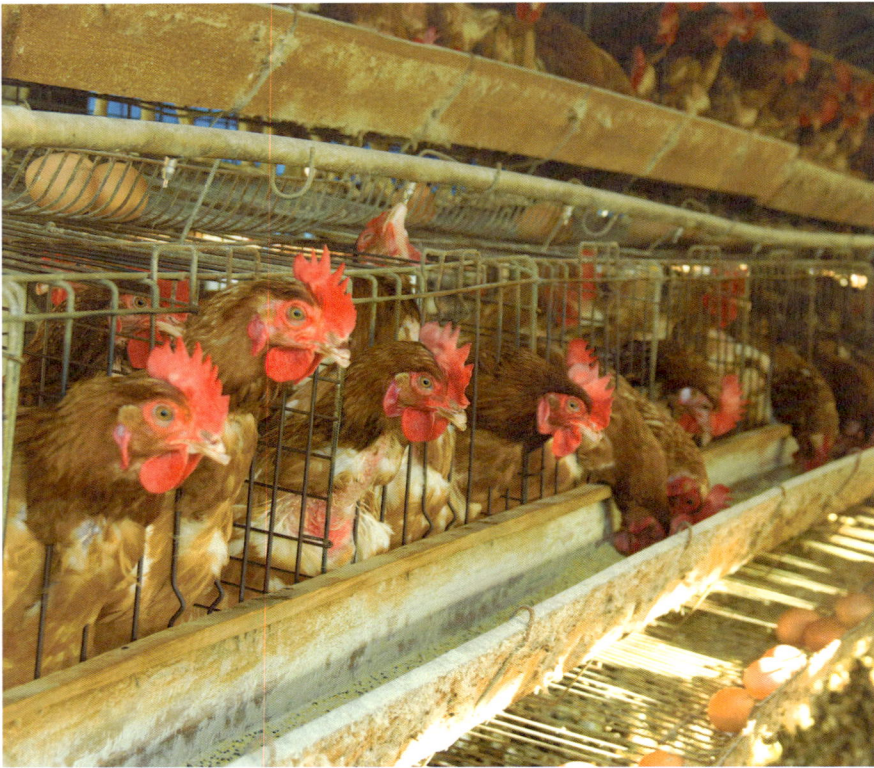

Most farm animals today don't live on green pastures.

Raising animals in crowded conditions, even cages, is more profitable. This type of farm is called a factory farm.

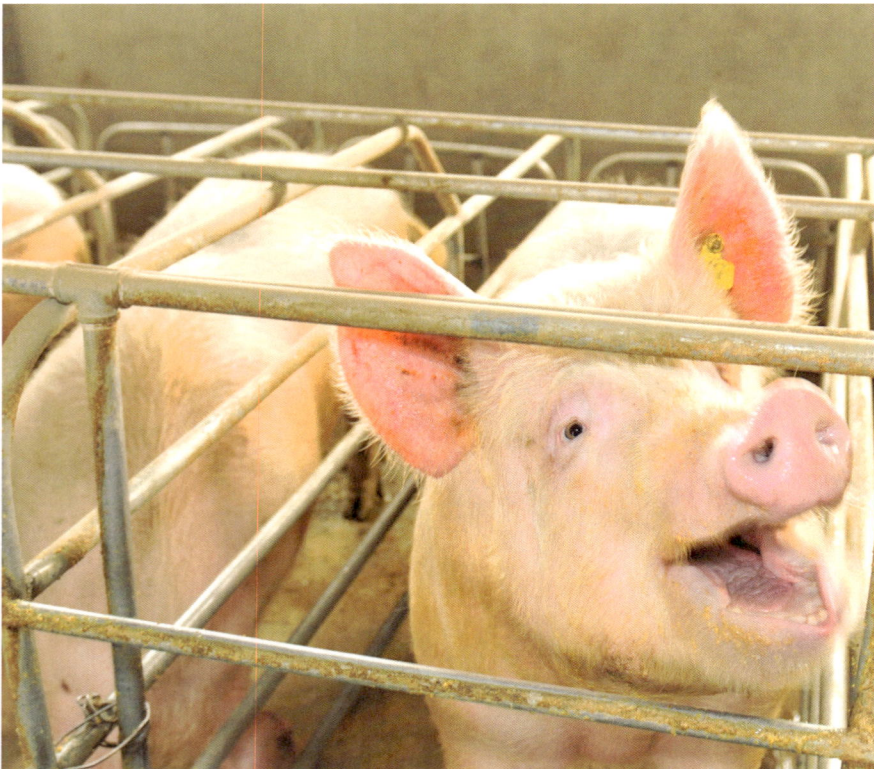

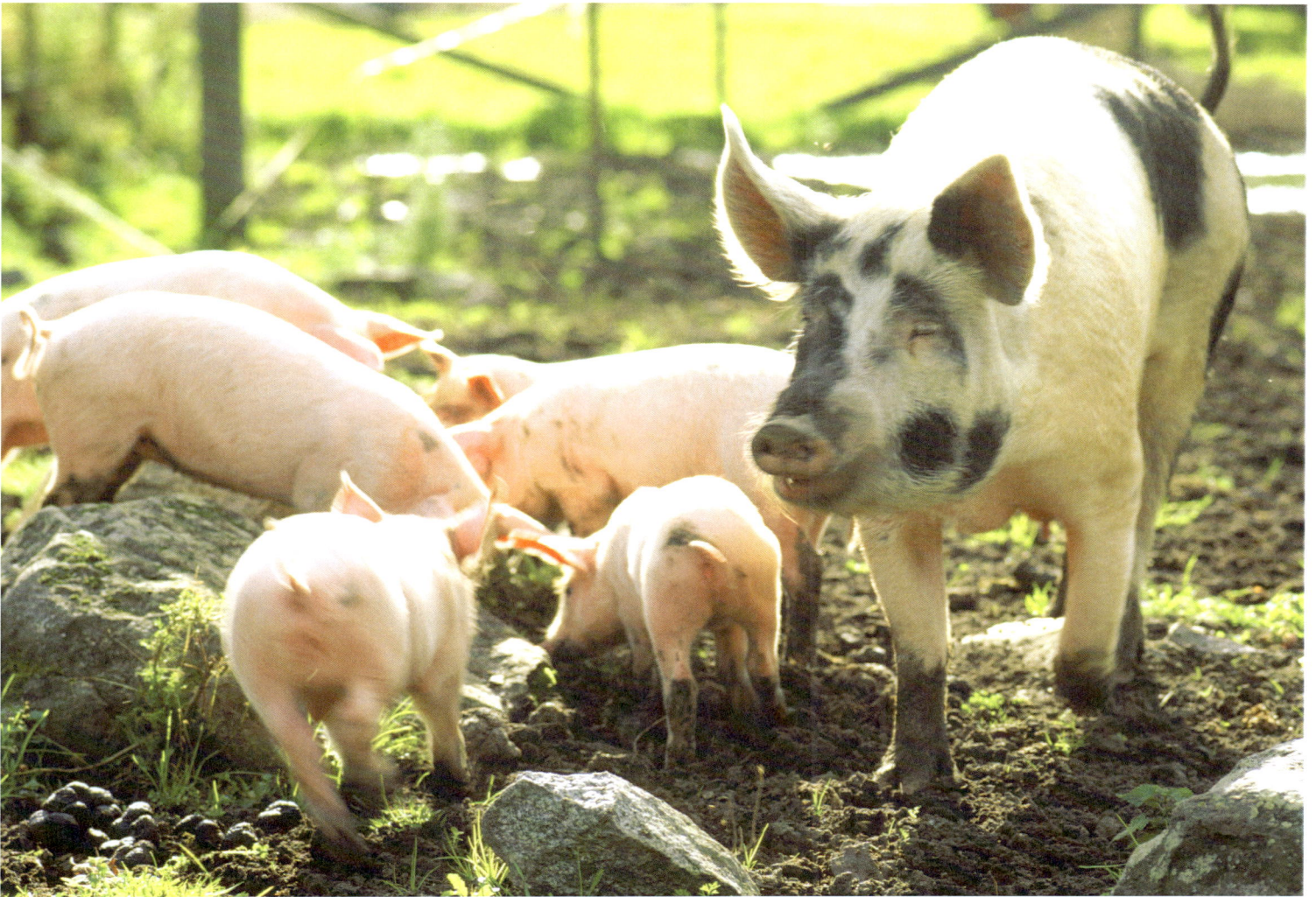

But as more and more people choose nuts and beans for plant-protein, less animals will need to be raised for food on unhappy factory-like farms.

All animals have feelings, and deserve to live happy and free!

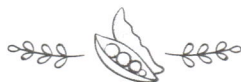

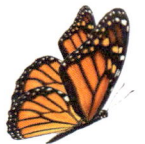

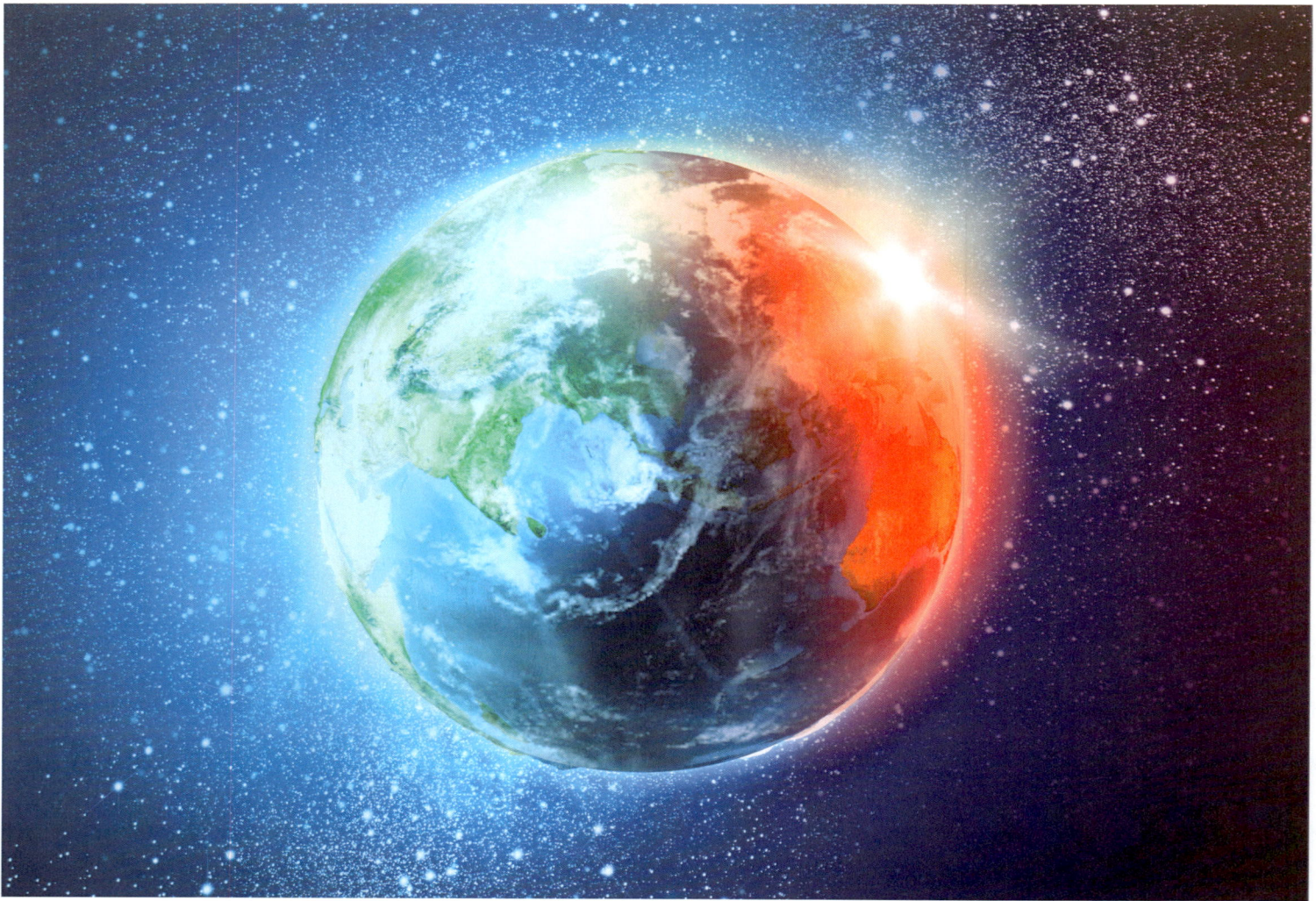

There's no place like home. For as far as the biggest telescope can see, looking out into the most far away galaxies, there is no other planet like Earth.

No other planet has oceans and rivers, amazing plants and beautiful animals - like you!

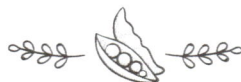

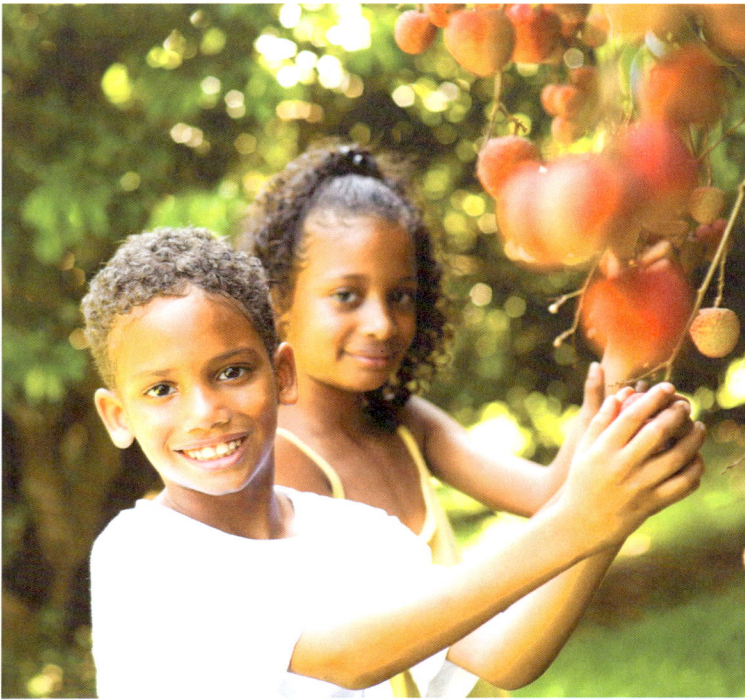
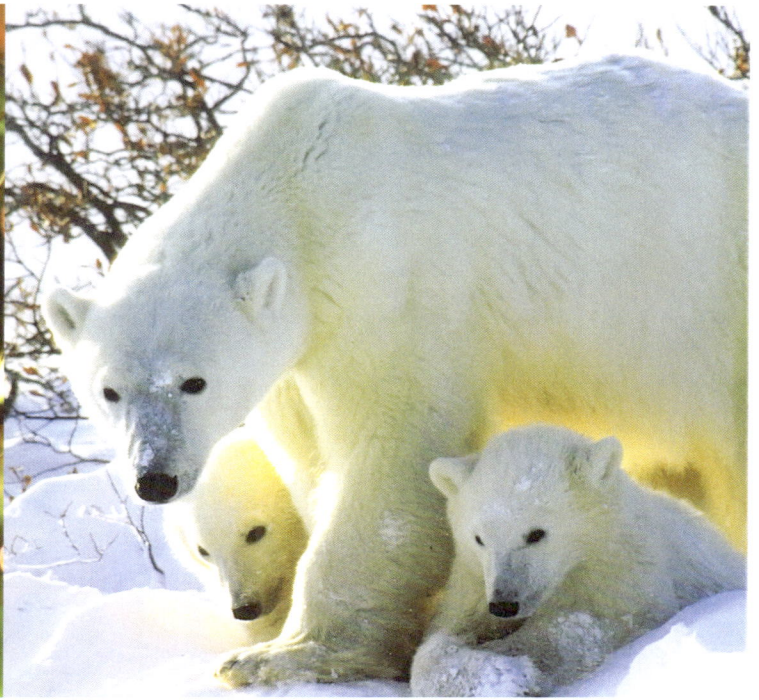

You have the super power to protect precious natural resources, precious animals, and your precious self everyday by eating *lean and green...*

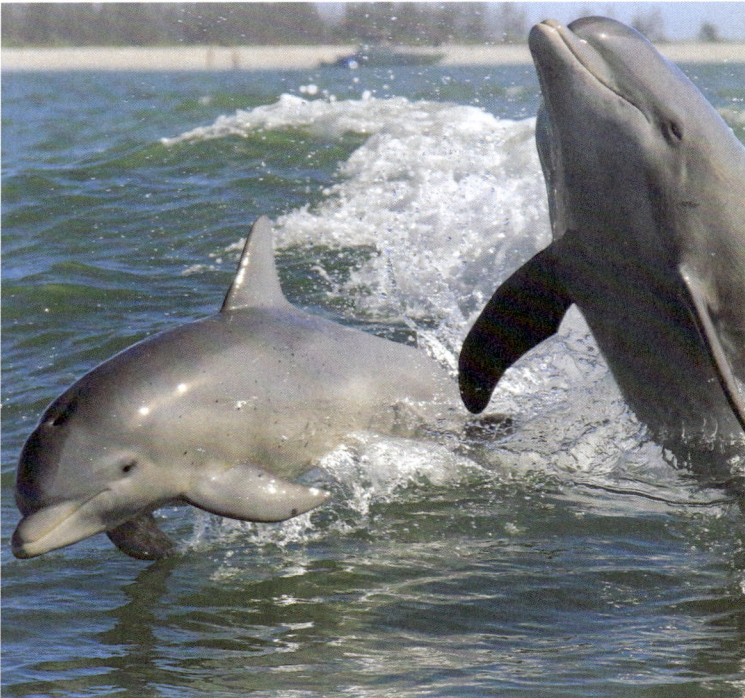
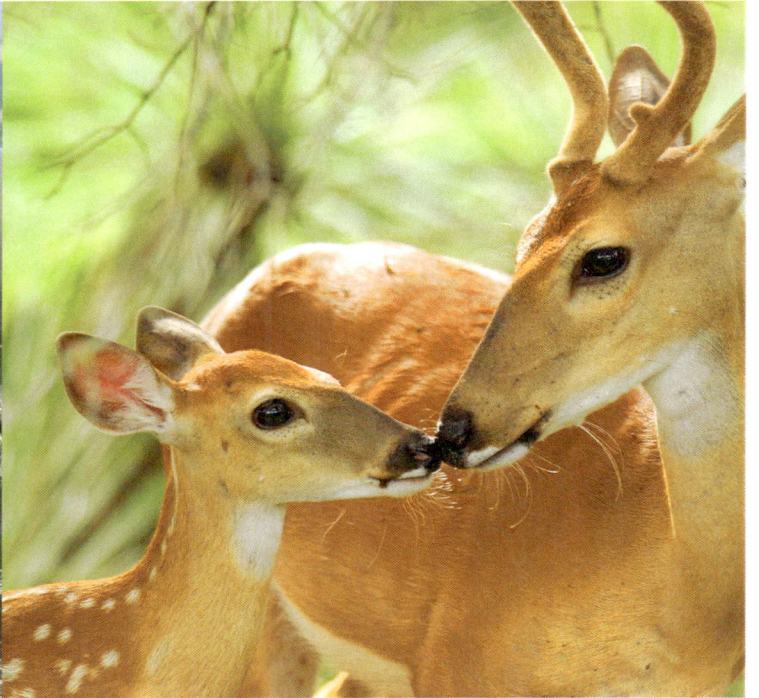

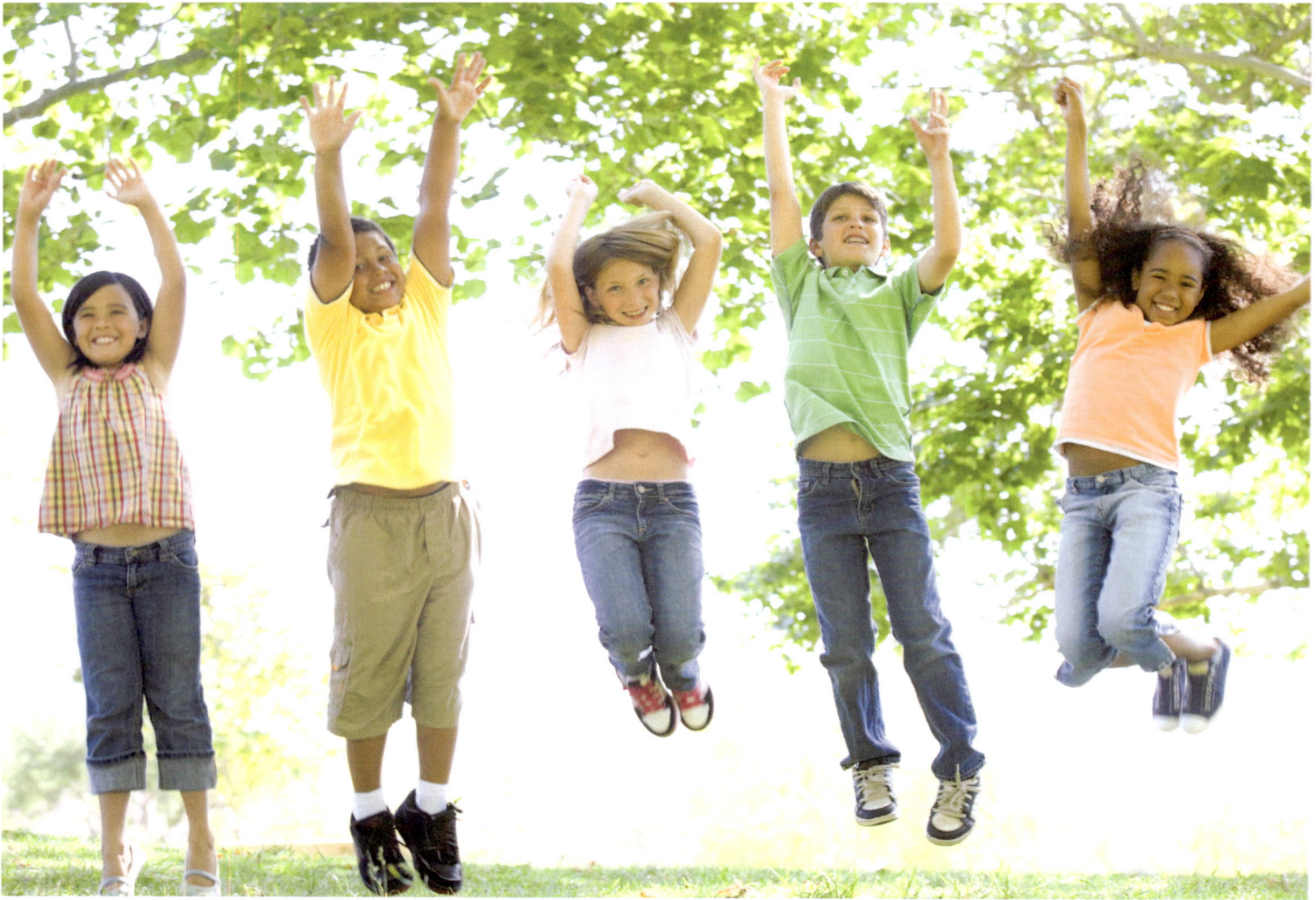

... with super foods to save the planet!

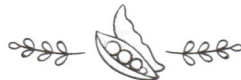

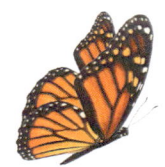

Afterword

A child's open heart and caring spirit can inspire us when we have become weary in a busy and complex world. Children renew our sense of wonder and appreciation for nature's gifts, including the nourishing food that grows from Earth's soil.

I wrote *Eating Lean and Green with Super Foods to Save the Planet!* to nurture that sense of wonder and care, and to empower children to protect our precious planet and their precious selves everyday with one simple action, healthful eating.

But if healthful eating was easy, everyone would be doing it. This book serves not only to educate children about smart food choices, but to approach nutrition education in a holistic way, with consideration for animals and the environment. This honest and integrative approach is the formula for meaningful and lasting change.

Every day, with each meal, we have an opportunity to co-create a healthier, greener and happier future for all. May our profound love of wondrous Earth, animals and each other be renewed everyday, and with every blessed meal.

All proceeds from the sale of this book benefit
Lean and Green Kids
a children's eco-health education & advocacy organization.

Check website for more educational resources (K-12) that meet common core standards and align with the principles in *Eating Lean and Green with Super Foods to Save the Planet!*
leanandgreenkids.org

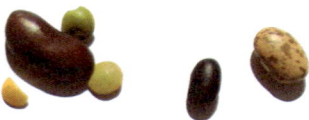

About the Author

Barbara Cole Gates
a.k.a. Queen Bean

When Barbara was a little girl, she loved nature and wanted to protect animals. She would find homes for stray animals and "relocate" spiders from inside her house to the remarkable outdoors.

As a mom and a teacher, Barbara wanted to protect children too. She learned that teaching good nutrition was a way to protect children, animals, and nature.

Barbara wrote *Eating Lean and Green* so she could help change the world into a healthier and happier place, one little bean at a time.

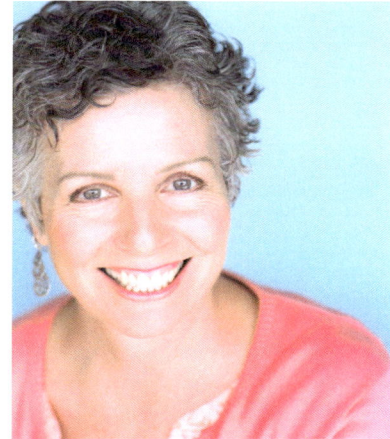

Also by Barbara Cole Gates
Jack and the Bean Stew

This book is a project of *Lean and Green Kids* and was made possible in part by the generous support of
Heal the Planet & A Well Fed World

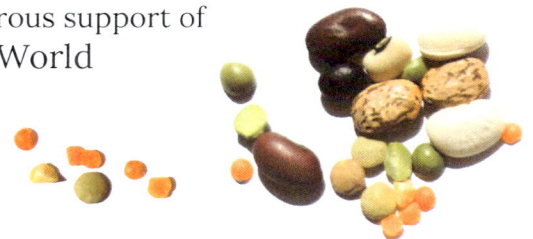

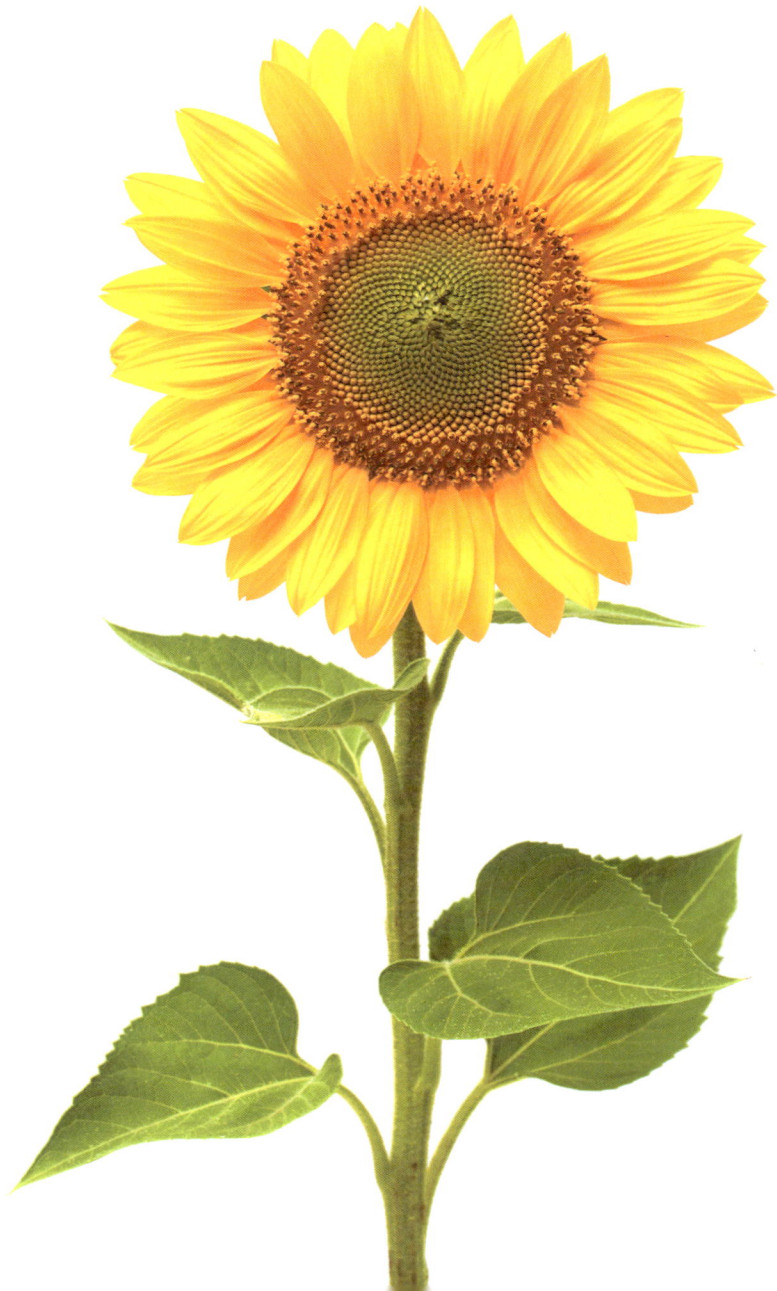

The hardest part of returning to a truly healthy environment may be changing the current totally unsustainable heavy-meat-eating culture of increasing numbers of people around the world.

But we must try.
We must make a start, one by one.

Jane Goodall

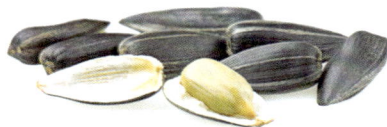

www.ingramcontent.com/pod-product-compliance
Lightning Source LLC
Chambersburg PA
CBRC101143030426
42336CB00008B/72